# OSCE Revision for the

# OSCE Revision for the Final FRCEM

**Rachel Goss** MBBS BSc (Hons) FRCEM

*Emergency Medicine Physician, Saint John Regional Hospital, New Brunswick*
*Assistant Professor, Department of Emergency Medicine, Dalhousie University, Canada*

**Emma McMaster** MBChB MMedSci BSc (Hons) FRCEM

*Emergency Medicine Consultant, University Hospital Plymouth, UK*

**Stephanie Rennie** BSc (Hons) MBBS MRCP (2013) FRCEM

*Emergency Medicine Consultant, Royal Cornwall Hospitals NHS Trust, UK*

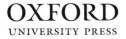

OXFORD
UNIVERSITY PRESS

# OXFORD
## UNIVERSITY PRESS

Great Clarendon Street, Oxford, OX2 6DP,
United Kingdom

Oxford University Press is a department of the University of Oxford.
It furthers the University's objective of excellence in research, scholarship,
and education by publishing worldwide. Oxford is a registered trade mark of
Oxford University Press in the UK and in certain other countries

© Oxford University Press 2021

The moral rights of the authors have been asserted

First Edition published in 2021

Published in the United States of America by Oxford University Press
198 Madison Avenue, New York, NY 10016, United States of America

British Library Cataloguing in Publication Data
Data available

Library of Congress Control Number: 2021933267

ISBN 978–0–19–885658–0

DOI: 10.1093/med/9780198856580.001.0001

Printed in Great Britain by
Bell & Bain Ltd., Glasgow

This book is dedicated to

*Dr Cliff Mann OBE, one of Emergency Medicines greatest leaders. An inspiring teacher, role model and mentor—may he Rest in Peace.*

# Foreword

I am delighted to introduce and recommend this examination revision text for the FRCEM OSCE examination.

Demonstrating clinical competence with a patient-centred approach in the OSCE examination via the integration of years of emergency department (ED) experience with a breadth and depth of knowledge is the pinnacle achievement for the aspiring emergency physician.

As a former President of the College, my happiest memories were the annual diploma ceremonies. Meeting so many successful candidates and their proud families was a genuine privilege. My delight at each and every success was underpinned by the knowledge that each candidate had been rigorously assessed in the examination.

This book provides an invaluable aid to revision for the FRCEM and will enable the candidate to use their preparation time both efficiently and effectively.

Each of the authors is a relatively recent successful candidate and so their insights and guidance are all the more relevant.

I wish all those preparing for the FRCEM the very best of fortune in their preparations—time spent revising from this book will undoubtedly be time well spent!

Dr C. J. Mann OBE FRCEM FRCP FRCA
Past President of the Royal College of Emergency Medicine

# Preface

The Objective Structured Clinical Examination (OSCE) is one of four components of the FRCEM Final Examination. Successful completion of the FRCEM Final Examination, along with achieving the training programme competencies, is a requirement to obtaining the Certificate of Completion of Training (CCT).

This book aims to equip the trainee with a solid approach to revision in order to pass the FRCEM OSCE. It outlines the structure and format of the exam, and provides useful tips on revision strategy and on how to navigate the exam on the day.

The chapters are divided into the different focus areas of the OSCE stations: history, examination, teaching skills, practical skills and procedures, communication skills, resuscitation scenarios, psychiatry cases, and management scenarios. The content is pertinent to the Royal College of Emergency Medicine (RCEM) curriculum and is based on best practice and up-to-date national guidance. Each chapter provides numerous OSCE scenarios with brief instructions for the candidate and clear mark schemes, as well as learning points for the trickier cases. Overall, this book provides a great structure for revision and the authors wish the candidates every success.

Rachel Goss
Emma McMaster
Stephanie Rennie

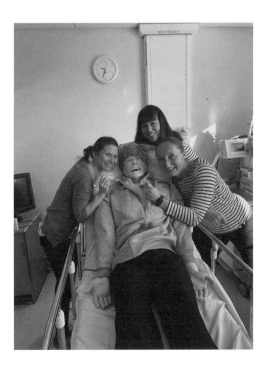

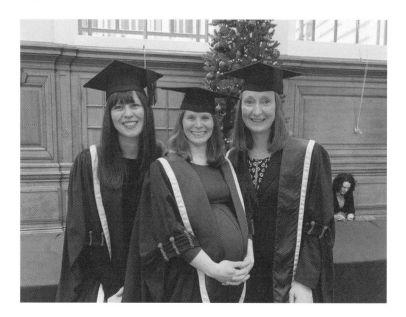

# Acknowledgements

We would like to say a very special thank you to each of our families. Their encouragement, support, and patience have been instrumental to our success in the FRCEM exams and the completion of this project.

# Contents

# Abbreviations

| | |
|---|---|
| AAA | abdominal aortic aneurysm |
| ABG | arterial blood gas |
| AC | air conduction |
| ACJ | acromioclavicular joint |
| ACP | advanced clinical practitioner |
| ACS | acute coronary syndrome |
| AF | atrial fibrillation |
| ALS | advanced life support |
| AOM | acute otitis media |
| AP | anteroposterior |
| APLS | advanced paediatric life support |
| ASIS | anterior superior iliac spine |
| ATLS | advanced trauma life support |
| AUDIT-C | Alcohol Use Disorders Identification Test |
| AXR | abdominal X-ray |
| BBV | blood-borne virus |
| BC | bone conduction |
| BD | twice daily |
| BIPAP | bilevel positive airway pressure |
| BMI | body mass index |
| BP | blood pressure |
| bpm | beats per minute |
| BPPV | benign paroxysmal positional vertigo |
| BTS | British Thoracic Society |
| BVM | bag–valve–mask |
| CCT | Certificate of Completion of Training |
| CES | cauda equina syndrome |
| CN | cranial nerve |
| CO2 | carbon dioxide |
| COCP | combined oral contraceptive pill |
| COPD | chronic obstructive pulmonary disease |
| COX-2 | cyclo-oxygenase |
| CPR | cardiopulmonary resuscitation |
| CRP | C-reactive protein |
| CRT | capillary refill time |
| C-spine | cervical spine |

| | |
|---|---|
| CT | computerised tomography |
| CTPA | computerised tomography pulmonary angiography |
| CXR | chest X-ray |
| DC | direct current |
| DCCV | direct current cardioversion |
| DDH | developmental dysplasia of the hip |
| DH | drug history |
| DKA | diabetic ketoacidosis |
| DSH | deliberate self-harm |
| DVLA | Driver and Vehicle Licensing Agency |
| DVT | deep vein thrombosis |
| EC | emergency contraception |
| ECG | electrocardiogram |
| ED | emergency department |
| ENP | emergency nurse practitioner |
| ENT | ear, nose, and throat |
| EPO | erythropoietin |
| ETCO2 | end-tidal carbon dioxide |
| ETT | endotracheal tube |
| F1 | Foundation Year 1 |
| F2 | Foundation Year 2 |
| FAST | focused assessment with sonography for trauma |
| FAST | Fast Alcohol Screening Test |
| FBC | full blood count |
| FDP | flexor digitorum profundus |
| FDS | flexor digitorum superficialis |
| FFP | fresh frozen plasma |
| FIB | fascia iliaca block |
| FOOSH | fall onto an outstretched hand |
| FPL | flexor pollicis longus |
| FRCEM | Fellowship of the Royal College of Emergency Medicine |
| G | gauge |
| GCS | Glasgow Coma Scale |
| GMC | General Medical Council |
| GP | general practitioner |
| GTN | glyceryl trinitrate |
| GU | genitourinary |
| GUM | genitourinary medicine |
| HDU | high dependency unit |

| | |
|---|---|
| HIV | human immunodeficiency virus |
| HMIMMS | Hospital Major Incident Management and Medical Support |
| HR | heart rate |
| HTN | hypertension |
| Hz | hertz |
| IJV | internal jugular vein |
| INR | international normalised ratio |
| IO | intraosseous |
| ITU | intensive therapy unit |
| IUD | intrauterine device |
| IV | intravenous |
| IVDU | intravenous drug user |
| J | joule |
| JVP | jugular venous pressure |
| kg | kilogram |
| kPa | kilopascal |
| LFT | liver function test |
| LLL | left lower lobe |
| LMN | lower motor neurone |
| LMP | last menstrual period |
| LUQ | left upper quadrant |
| m | metre |
| MCA | Mental Capacity Act |
| MCPJ | metacarpophalangeal joint |
| mg | milligram |
| MHA | mental health assessment |
| MIU | minor injuries unit |
| ml | millilitre |
| MMSE | Mini-Mental State Examination |
| mph | miles per hour |
| MRC | Medical Research Council |
| MRCEM | Membership of the Royal College of Emergency Medicine |
| MRI | magnetic resonance imaging |
| MTC | major trauma centre |
| NAD | nicotinamide adenine dinucleotide |
| NAI | non-accidental injury |
| NICE | National Institute for Health and Care Excellence |
| NLS | newborn life support |
| NSAID | non-steroidal anti-inflammatory drug |

| | |
|---|---|
| O2 | oxygen |
| OCP | oral contraceptive pill |
| OD | once daily |
| ORIF | open reduction and internal fixation |
| OSCE | Objective Structured Clinical Examination |
| PALS | Patient Advice and Liaison Service |
| PAT | Paddington Alcohol Test |
| PE | pulmonary embolism |
| PEA | pulseless electrical activity |
| PEP | post-exposure prophylaxis |
| PERC | Pulmonary Embolism Rule-out Criteria |
| PEWS | Paediatric Early Warning Score |
| PIPJ | proximal interphalangeal joint |
| PMR | polymyalgia rheumatica |
| PO | per os (oral) |
| PPE | personal protective equipment |
| PPH | post-partum haemorrhage |
| PPM | permanent pacemaker |
| PR | per rectum |
| PRN | as needed |
| PV | per vaginum |
| PXR | pelvic X-ray |
| RAPD | relative afferent pupillary defect |
| RCEM | Royal College of Emergency Medicine |
| RIF | right iliac fossa |
| ROSC | return of spontaneous circulation |
| RR | respiratory rate |
| RSI | rapid sequence induction |
| SaO2 | oxygen saturation of arterial blood |
| SEM | standard error of measurement |
| SHO | Senior House Officer |
| SNOD | specialist nurse for organ donation |
| SOB | shortness of breath; short of breath |
| SOL | space-occupying lesion |
| SpR | specialty registrar |
| SSRI | selective serotonin reuptake inhibitor |
| ST1 | Specialty Trainee Year 1 |
| ST2 | Specialty Trainee Year 2 |
| ST3 | Specialty Trainee Year 3 |

| | |
|---|---|
| STEMI | ST-elevation myocardial infarction |
| STI | sexually transmitted infection |
| SUFE | slipped upper femoral epiphysis |
| TDS | three times daily |
| TIA | transient ischaemic attack |
| TLOC | transient loss of consciousness |
| TMJ | temporomandibular joint |
| TTL | trauma team leader |
| TURBT | transurethral resection of bladder tumour |
| TXA | tranexamic acid |
| U&E | urea and electrolytes |
| UMN | upper motor neurone |
| UPSI | unprotected sexual intercourse |
| USS | ultrasound scan |
| UTI | urinary tract infection |
| VA | visual acuity |
| VF | ventricular fibrillation |
| VT | ventricular tachycardia |
| VTE | venous thromboembolism |
| VZIG | varicella-zoster immunoglobulin |

# Chapter 1 **The FRCEM OSCE**

Passing the Fellowship of the Royal College of Emergency Medicine (FRCEM) Objective Structured Clinical Examination (OSCE) is a very achievable feat. It is a fair exam that really does just feel like a busy day at work. The FRCEM exam scenarios and topics may be similar to those in the Membership of the Royal College of Emergency Medicine (MRCEM) OSCE, but the fellowship exam is designed to assess candidates at a more senior level; therefore, more leadership, management, and conflict resolution skills are required. This textbook aims to prepare and test these key skills.

This book has been written by three UK-trained Emergency Medicine Consultants as a revision aid, designed to prepare you for the final FRCEM OSCE. It provides an invaluable guide to the structure and format of the exam, as well as covering the core topics that are examined. We have provided example OSCEs with mark sheets, as well as candidate, examiner, and actor information and lists of equipment required.

We hope that you will find this book not only a useful revision aid, but also a helpful guide to obtaining the required skills to transition into a new consultant.

# Before the Exam: Revision Strategy

We, the authors, revised as a group. It is important to have a buddy with whom to practise. You need to work through scenarios in real time, with your buddy scoring and timing you. It is very difficult to prepare for this exam on your own. Try and get your department to run some simulations or stations for you and be watched day to day by as many people as possible.

It is really important to practise against the clock. You will be surprised by how quickly the time goes by, especially in the history stations and the stations where you need to leave time to discuss a management plan at the end.

Think through any potential stations as a group and figure out what the key marks would be and how you will achieve these.

Familiarise yourself with the latest Royal College of Emergency Medicine (RCEM) guidance and examination guidelines available on the RCEM website.

We booked several sessions in our hospital's simulation suite and went through the typical Advanced Life Support (ALS), Advanced Paediatric Life Support (APLS), and Advanced Trauma Life Support (ATLS) scenarios. As we mention in Chapter 7 in resuscitation scenarios, the OSCE resuscitation stations are no harder than those encountered on the above courses. However, there will be additional marks for another element such as communication, a practical procedure, or teaching. We recommend you work through the scenarios from these courses, but make them as hard as you can, bouncing between different arrhythmias and types of cardiac arrest. By doing this, you will have covered everything they can throw at you and more!

If you have time, attend or teach on the life support courses.

We recommend you work through the scenarios in this book and the lists of possible stations we have provided in a group. Mark each other harshly and provide honest feedback. Learn the generic marks common to each type of scenario and be able to adapt them to any variation of the station.

This book is not intended to be a complete textbook, but a resource to use as a building block which will allow you to approach any station and get the core marks, and to provide you with a strategy to pass with a good mark.

The clinical and management aspects of the stations are based on guidelines correct at the time of writing. Emergency medicine is a fast-paced specialty, so be aware of the latest guidelines and current thinking.

As is true to medicine, there is not always an absolute right or wrong answer. For example, in a station requiring a rapid sequence induction (RSI), the mark sheet will not have a specific list of RSI drugs and doses that you must use. If you say something sensible, you will get the marks. Do what you would do at work!

The examiners do get fatigued. Speak loudly and clearly, and be as engaging as you can. If you make a good impression and come across as someone safe and competent who seems to know what they are talking about, you may well be given the benefit of the doubt if the examiner missed a key point you mentioned.

You should wear scrubs or smart professional attire to the exam. Be comfortable, be bare below the elbows, and look professional. Do not turn up in filthy, garish trainers or scrubs that have been screwed up in your gym bag for a month. You can take your stethoscope with you. You would be expected to use the appropriate personal protective equipment for any face to face patient interaction or procedure.

# In the Exam

Walk in confidently and introduce yourself to the patient; be polite and, if needed, recap any information that you have been given outside the room.

You are expected to perform at the level of a new consultant on their first day at work. The College uses the simulated clinical scenarios to assess whether candidates have sufficient clinical knowledge and skills to gain the Certificate of Completion of Training (CCT) as an Emergency Medicine Consultant.

The exam consists of sixteen 8-minute stations, two of which are double resuscitation stations and two are rest stations. You have one minute to read the instructions before entering the room.

This one minute must be used wisely. Not only do you need to read and digest the instructions, but you also need to review the pie chart. It is not always clear from the instructions what the focus of the station is. The pie chart gives you key information you need, so that you can tell the main focus of the station. You do not want to take a full history when actually the station wanted a focused history and discussion about management or breaking bad news.

This time can also be used to think about key marks that you need to gain in the room. For example, thinking through the pertinent questions for a history station, the relevant points in a teaching station, the resus algorithm you are likely to need, or calculating the weight for a WETFLAG. Make sure you can fluently calculate a WETFLAG under pressure. We recommend you calculate the weight and arrest dose for intravenous (IV) adrenaline outside the room, which then also provides you with the dose for lorazepam.

# Example Station

## Instructions for the Candidate

A 56-year-old man presents with haematuria and urinary retention. He has already had a catheter inserted and is more comfortable. His general practitioner (GP) referred him for a computerised tomography (CT) scan recently, as he has been complaining of flank pain and haematuria. The patient has not yet received these results, but they are available to you. Please discuss the ongoing management plan with the patient.

## Mark Scheme Breakdown

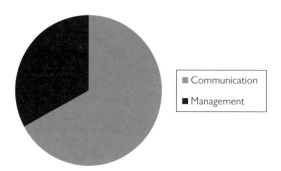

**Figure 1.1** Example station mark scheme breakdown.

You might read the information outside the room and think that the station requires a brief history and then a management plan regarding catheter removal and catheter care. However, when you look at the pie chart, you will see that the marks are weighted more towards communication. You will need a brief summary of the patient's symptoms and what information the GP has given them regarding a possible diagnosis and why a CT was performed. You need to notice that the candidate information tells you the results are available to you. You will need to read and digest these in the room. This should then shift your focus towards breaking bad news. The patient actually has a new cancer diagnosis with a suspected renal cell carcinoma. You will need to focus the scenario on breaking bad news, as well as inform the patient of what the follow-up plan will be regarding catheter care, urology/oncology, etc.

Read the candidate information very carefully as it is easy to go off on the wrong track. We recommend you read it twice and then summarise the information to the patient where appropriate. Take cues from the patient; they may try and guide you if you are on the wrong track. If you need to, take a pause and ask to read the candidate information again if things do not seem to be going well.

In some stations, you will finish early. This may feel awkward, but the examiner will sit there in silence and not make conversation. If whilst you are sitting there, you think of another question or have another point to make, ask it! Although it is best if a history looks slick and is asked in a logical order, adding in a question after a pause is fine and will still get you the mark. Use this time wisely to think through any marks you may have missed, and to reset for the next station.

When the bell goes, thank those involved in the station and leave promptly and proceed to the next station. Do not dwell on how the previous station went; focus on the station you are now entering.

The final mark is cumulative for all stations, so if the last station went badly, move on and focus on making up the marks as you move forward.

The curriculum areas assessed within the FRCEM Final OSCE are shown in Table 1.1.

**Table 1.1** FRCEM final OSCE curriculum areas

| Station | Curriculum area |
| --- | --- |
| 1 | Core acute |
| 2a | Resuscitation |
| 2b | Resuscitation |
| 3 | Core major |
| 4 | Common competences |
| 5 | Common competences |
| 6 | Anaesthetic competences |
| 7a | Paediatric resuscitation |
| 7b | Paediatric resuscitation |
| 8 | Paediatric acute |
| 9 | Paediatric major |
| 10 | HST major |
| 11 | HST and adult acute |
| 12 | Practical skills |
| 13 | Paediatric practical skills |
| 14 | Non-technical skills |

HST, higher specialty training.

# After the Exam

After the exam, you will receive your score and feedback broken down by question and topic. You will be given your score, the pass mark, and the average score, as well as a cumulative score and pass mark.

For simplicity, we have assigned one mark to each point on the mark sheet in this book. However, in the exam, up to three marks can be available for each point. Simple/binary points will be worth one mark, but more complex explanations can be worth two or three marks. For example, explaining successfully to a patient the diagnosis or management plan is likely to be worth three marks, yet asking a simple history question will be worth only one mark. One mark will be given for introducing yourself appropriately, confirming the patient's identity, and explaining the purpose of the consultation. More important complex points will be worth more marks. For example, explaining a procedure, such as inserting a chest drain during a resuscitation scenario, or the nature of a disease or the rationale for specific medications is likely to be worth more than one mark. In general, the mark sheets are out of 15 in the exam. We have given you more detailed mark sheets with one mark per point to aid in teaching key points you should be aware of.

The FRCEM Final OSCE is standard set using the borderline regression method. One standard error of measurement (SEM) will be added to the cut score identified using the borderline regression method to calculate the final pass mark. There are no critical sudden death stations. The pass mark is cumulative, so it is OK to have a terrible station and a few borderline ones; just make sure you reset and maximise marks on the other stations.

A maximum of four attempts is allowed.

The RCEM curriculum will be updated in 2021. Whilst the format may be different and new items may be added to the curriculum, we believe it is unlikely that a significant amount of the current curriculum will be removed. We expect that the example stations and generic mark schemes will remain useful and relevant despite potential changes in the curriculum, as they are based on core topics and up-to-date guidance.

Practise, practise, practise.

Good luck!

Most of all, enjoy your revision. It is a good feeling to know you are at the peak of your knowledge and to feel able to cope with any scenario, be it in real life or in an exam.

# Chapter 2 **History and Management**

# The History and Management Station

The FRCEM OSCE is an opportunity to put into practice all that you have learnt during your training so far. This chapter challenges you to combine your history-taking and communication skills and your knowledge of current guidelines to assess a patient and agree on an appropriate management plan with them. You can often expect an added nuance to the station that requires you to go beyond simply taking a history and use your skills of negotiation, de-escalation, and advanced communication, just as you do in real life.

Use the pie chart to see what the focus of the station is and apportion your time accordingly. Use the information provided in the question. There may be investigation results or referral letters available to you. Use clinical scoring tools and guidelines relevant to the presenting complaint to steer your questions and management plan. Do not worry if you ask a question out of the conventional order—it is better to ask it late than not at all.

Time yourself so that you can gauge how long it takes to complete the station and then hone your technique to ensure you are within the time limit. Keep going until you know how long eight minutes 'feels'. You will create your own routine where some questions can be rapidly ticked off, while others need more time and sensitivity.

Finally, keep practising. Practise on your own, with your study buddies, with your family, or even with your teddy bear. It will be worth it.

## 2.1   Chickenpox

### Instructions for Candidate

Please take a history and discuss the management with the mother of a child who has a vesicular rash.

### Mark Scheme Breakdown

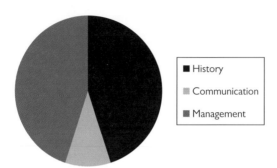

**Figure 2.1.1**  Chickenpox mark scheme breakdown.

### Instructions for Actor

You are the mother of a five-year-old girl with vesicular rash. She is systemically well and the rash is moderate. She has no past medical history, is well, and is eating and drinking.

You are also 36/40 weeks pregnant. You are uncertain if you have had chickenpox before. You have no idea that chickenpox in pregnancy has implications to the baby. You live with your husband who has just received his last cycle of chemotherapy for testicular cancer.

### Instructions for Examiner

Provide the candidate with an image of the vesicular rash (Fig. 2.1.2).

### Equipment Required

Image of chickenpox rash (Fig. 2.1.2).

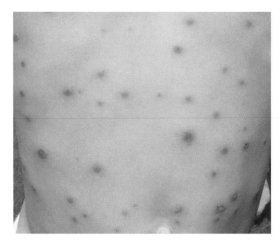

**Figure 2.1.2** Chickenpox rash.

(from Fig 9.16A Dermatology, from Training in Paediatrics by Mark Gardiner, Sarah Eisen, and Catherine Murphy. Oxford University Press. ISBN 9780199227730)

## Mark Scheme

| | |
|---|---|
| Introduces self to mother and child | |
| Asks an open question regarding reason for attendance | |
| Asks to see rash (photo provided) | |
| Confirms key details in history for child: | |
| • Onset of rash | |
| • Systemic symptoms: fever/level of activity | |
| • Fluid status | |
| • Urine output | |
| • Previous episodes | |
| Past medical history: specifically confirms child is not immunocompromised, has no significant cardiorespiratory disease, and has no chronic skin disorders | |
| Drug history: including when last doses of paracetamol/ibuprofen were given | |
| Immunisation status | |
| Perinatal history | |
| Social history: it is key to know who else is in the house (immunocompromised husband) | |

| | |
|---|---|
| Confirm mother is pregnant: | |
| • Gestation | |
| • Previous history of chickenpox | |
| Maternal past medical history, drug history, immunisations, and brief obstetric history | |
| **Child:** | |
| • States they will need to fully examine the child and get a set of observations | |
| • Assuming she is well and the observations are normal, they can go home | |
| • Advice on regular paracetamol and avoiding ibuprofen | |
| • Safety net advice if fluid input and urine output reduce | |
| • Advises about signs of secondary infection | |
| • Advises she is infectious for two days before rash to six days afterwards or once crusted over; therefore, five days' exclusion from school and the need to isolate from pregnant mothers or neonates | |
| • Advises regarding red flags and provides safety net to return | |
| **Mother:** | |
| • Confirms she is asymptomatic | |
| • If she does not know her chickenpox status, offers a varicella-zoster virus immunoglobulin (VZIG) blood test to confirm | |
| • Explains if she is immune, no treatment is required | |
| • Explains if she is not immune, VZIG can be given (up to ten days after exposure) | |
| **Father:** | |
| • Enquires whether he has had significant exposure to the child (face-to-face/>15 minutes) | |
| • Confirms whether he is immunocompromised | |
| • Advises he seeks medical attention via GP/oncologist as likely to need treatment | |
| • Advises separating father and child whilst child is still infectious | |
| Explores ideas, concerns, and expectations and asks if they have any questions | |
| Summarises consultation | |
| Demonstrates good communication and addresses mother's concerns | |

Total    **/34**

## Learning Points

*Risks of Chickenpox in Pregnancy*

First trimester: no increased risk of miscarriage.

Second trimester: small risk of foetal varicella syndrome (2.8%).

Third trimester: if contracted in the last four weeks of pregnancy, there is a risk of newborn infection. Ideally, avoid delivery for seven days after the rash. If the baby is born fewer than seven days from the onset of the rash, or the mother develops clinical varicella within 28 days of delivery, give VZIG to the neonate.

In this case, if the mother at 36/40 gestation did have a chickenpox rash, treatment would be recommended:

- If <24 hours since first lesion appeared and >20/40, give oral (PO) aciclovir 500 mg five times per day for seven days. Discharge home with safety net advice.
- If >24 hours since the first lesion appeared and she has severe disease (respiratory involvement/neurological involvement/haemorrhagic rash/dense mucosal rash) or is immunocompromised, has chronic lung disease, is a smoker, or has >100 lesions, admit for IV aciclovir.

## References

https://cks.nice.org.uk/chickenpox
https://www.rcog.org.uk/globalassets/documents/guidelines/gtg13.pdf

## 2.2 **Cervical Spine Assessment**

### Instructions for Candidate

Please take a history and discuss the management with this patient who has been involved in a road traffic collision and now has neck pain. The patient is deaf but can lip-read and speak clearly.

### Mark Scheme Breakdown

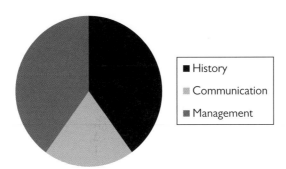

**Figure 2.2.1** Cervical spine mark scheme breakdown.

### Instructions for Actor

You are a 34-year-old male who was the passenger in a stationary car which was rear-ended two hours ago. You were stopped at traffic lights when another car travelling at approximately 20 mph hit into the back of your car. You got out of the vehicle yourself and felt fine on the scene. You have walked into the emergency department (ED) but have since developed pain in your neck. You have been given some paracetamol at triage but are still sore. You have never had any previous neck problems. You are concerned you have broken something and are keen for an X-ray. When the doctor explains why you do not need an X-ray, you accept this and ask for analgesia to take home.

You are deaf but can lip-read if the doctor faces you and speaks clearly. You can speak and respond clearly. If they do not face you, you cannot understand them and will not give information.

### Instructions for Examiner

Observation only.

### Equipment Required

None.

## Mark Scheme

| | |
|---|---|
| Introduces self to patient | |
| Asks an open question regarding reason for attendance | |
| Recognises the patient is deaf, offers an interpreter, and assesses the best form of communication | |
| Offers further analgesia | |
| Confirms key points from history: | |
| • Mechanism (confirms low-risk mechanism: simple rear-end shunt) | |
| • Seat belt worn and head rest in car | |
| • Self-extricated, mobile since accident/sitting in ED | |
| • Time of accident | |
| • When did the neck pain start? Location of pain? Severity? Character? | |
| • Paraesthesia or weakness in limbs | |
| • Previous neck disease/injury/surgery | |
| • Is Glasgow Coma Scale (GCS) 15/not intoxicated | |
| Past medical history | |
| Drug history and allergies | |
| Social history | |
| Explains the need to examine the patient to assess for midline tenderness, perform a peripheral nerve exam, and assess neck movement | |
| Assuming the examination is normal, you do not need to X-ray | |
| Explains why they do not need an X-ray | |
| Advises regarding discharge, regular analgesia, mobilising neck, and what to expect | |
| Checks understanding and asks if there are any specific concerns or questions | |

Total    /**20**

## Learning Points

### Canadian C-spine Rules

The Canadian C-spine rules are applicable to patients who have a GCS 15 and are haemodynamically stable and over 16 years, who have sustained trauma.

If the patient is >65 years, has paraesthesia in their extremities, or has been involved in a dangerous mechanism (examples include a fall >1 m or five steps, an axial load, a rollover or ejection from a vehicle, or involved in a motorised recreation vehicle/bicycle or horse), imaging is recommended.

If the patient has none of these features, was involved in a low-risk mechanism (simple rear-end motor vehicle collision), has been sitting in the ED, is ambulatory, and has delayed-onset pain and no midline tenderness, they can be assessed clinically.

Clinical assessment: palpate for midline tenderness; assess power and sensation; ask to rotate the head 45° to the left and right.

Discharge with advice if the examination is normal.

# Reference

https://www.nice.org.uk/guidance/ng41/resources/spinal-injury-assessment-and-initial-management-pdf-1837447790533

## 2.3 **Atraumatic Knee Swelling**

### Instructions for Candidate

A 21-year-old man presents with a swollen knee. Take a history and explain the management plan. You do not need to examine the knee.

### Mark Scheme Breakdown

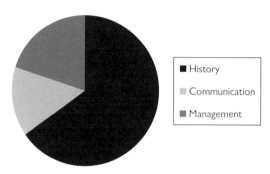

**Figure 2.3.1** Atraumatic knee swelling mark scheme breakdown.

### Instructions for Actor

You are a 21-year-old shoe shop assistant. The knee became swollen very quickly this morning. There was no injury that you can recollect. No other joints are affected and this has not happened before. You have haemophilia (type A—moderate/severe) and take factor VIII three times a week as prophylaxis. You have taken your medications today but could not get hold of your haematology team, so you came to the ED.

If asked, you are concerned about how you will manage at work as there is a lot of kneeling. You ask if the blood can be drained off from your knee and whether this episode will cause any long-term disability.

### Instructions for Examiner

Observation only.

### Equipment Required

None.

# Mark Scheme

| | |
|---|---|
| Introduces self to patient | |
| Offers analgesia | |
| Asks an open question to assess presenting complaint | |
| Asks about: | |
| • Timing | |
| • Injury | |
| • Other joints affected | |
| • Pain | |
| • Previous episodes | |
| • Fever | |
| • Systemic symptoms | |
| • Bleeding from anywhere else (gums/urine/bruising, etc.) | |
| Past medical history | |
| Establishes haemophilia and type | |
| Checks severity (mild/moderate/severe) | |
| Checks current management/treatment plan | |
| Drug history and allergies | |
| Social history | |
| Family history | |
| Explains the likely diagnosis | |
| Explains management plan: blood tests, discussion with haematology and orthopaedics | |
| Explains will need treatment with factors | |
| Answers the patient's questions where possible: not suitable for knee aspiration | |
| Advises the patient to avoid kneeling/trauma | |
| Informs the patient from where to get further help and advice if required | |
| Explores ideas, concerns, and expectations and asks if there are any further questions | |

Total    /**25**

## Learning Points

Early management strategies for acute haemarthrosis in haemophiliacs include:

- Analgesia: stepwise, paracetamol, selective cyclo-oxygenase 2 (COX-2) non-steroidal anti-inflammatory drugs (NSAIDs), then opioids.
- Rest: should continue until all clinical symptoms of haemarthrosis have resolved.
- Ice: crushed ice or ice packs can alleviate pain and swelling.
- Compression and elevation.
- Discussion with haematology about a factor VIII dosing strategy; a severe bleed may require a 12-hourly dosing schedule.
- Tranexamic acid is also useful, particularly for patients who have developed inhibitors.

The natural history of arthropathy in severe haemophilia is well described, with recurrent bleeds into joints leading to progressive joint damage and ultimate destruction, with associated functional problems. However, the early use of treatment with factor VIII in severe bleeds such as this one can potentially prevent/reduce permanent damage and avoid the cycle of damage associated with recurrent haemarthrosis.

Joint aspiration is not routinely recommended unless there is concern about septic arthritis. It may be useful for pain relief in tense haemarthrosis under appropriate haemostatic therapy.

## Reference

http://www.ukhcdo.org/wp-content/uploads/2017/03/Guidelines-for-the-management-of-acute-joint-bleeds-and-chronic-synovitis-in-haemophilia.pdf

## 2.4 **Croup**

### Instructions for Candidate

Please take a history and discuss the management with the mother of a child with respiratory distress. You do not need to examine the patient, but you may ask for key examination findings.

### Mark Scheme Breakdown

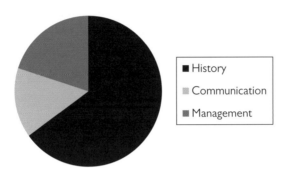

**Figure 2.4.1** Croup mark scheme breakdown.

### Instructions for Actor

You are the mother of a 12-month-old girl who has presented tonight with rapid breathing, intercostal recession, a cough, and a snotty nose. She has been coryzal for two days and her breathing has worsened overnight. She has had a temperature of 38°C, but this settled with paracetamol. Her food and drink intake has reduced since yesterday and she only managed to drink 50 ml and had two wet nappies yesterday. The baby has had no apnoea (absence of breathing) or cyanosis (blue lips/skin), is not floppy, and has had no grunting. She has no past medical history and was born at term by uncomplicated vaginal delivery. You are a smoker. If asked, you disclose that you have a difficult social situation as you are on your own and have no car; you cannot afford taxis to the hospital and cannot afford to buy any paracetamol this week.

### Instructions for Examiner

Give examination findings when asked: oxygen ($O_2$) saturations 94% in room air, respiratory rate (RR) 40, temperature 37.4°C, alert, barking cough, no wheeze, and mild intercostal recessions. The patient has successfully completed an oral fluid challenge in the department.

### Equipment Required

None.

## Mark Scheme

| | |
|---|---|
| Introduces self to mother and child | |
| Asks an open question regarding the reason for attendance | |
| Confirms key details in history for child: | |
| • Onset of symptoms | |
| • Systemic symptoms: fever/level of activity | |
| • Fluid status | |
| • Urine output | |
| • Cough | |
| • Coryzal | |
| • Work of breathing: grunting/nasal flare/recessions/tracheal tug | |
| • Apnoea | |
| • Cyanosis | |
| • Previous episodes | |
| Past medical history, specifically chronic lung disease/neuromuscular disorders | |
| Drug history (including recent doses of paracetamol/ibuprofen) and allergies | |
| Immunisation status | |
| Perinatal history | |
| Social history | |
| • Housing situation | |
| • Smoking in the house | |
| • Social support | |
| • Childcare setting | |
| States would like to examine the child—key examination findings will be given if asked for: | |
| • Activity/level of consciousness | |
| • RR and $O_2$ saturations | |
| • Assessment of work of breathing | |
| • Temperature | |
| • Heart rate (HR) | |
| Summary to parent of findings and diagnosis of croup | |

| | |
|---|---|
| Discusses admission or longer period of observation due to social situation, lack of support, and ongoing mild symptoms | |
| Addresses key questions/areas of concern | |
| If decides to discharge, discusses red flags and when to return:<br>• <50% fluids<br>• No wet nappies for 12 hours<br>• Signs of respiratory distress: explain to look for grunting/recessions/tachypnoea<br>• Exhaustion | |
| Advises not to smoke | |
| Answers mum's questions, good rapport | |

Total    /**31**

## Learning Points

Clinical classification of severity—as per National Institute for Health and Care Excellence (NICE) guidance:

**Mild**—barking cough, but no stridor or sternal/intercostal recession at rest.

**Moderate**—barking cough with stridor and sternal recession at rest; no agitation or lethargy.

**Severe**—barking cough with stridor and sternal/intercostal recession associated with agitation or lethargy.

**Impending respiratory failure**—increasing upper airway obstruction, sternal/intercostal recession, asynchronous chest wall and abdominal movement, fatigue, pallor or cyanosis, decreased level of consciousness, or tachycardia.

The Westley croup score is a commonly used tool which may be used to assess severity and thus guide management of the child. A total score of ≤1 is considered mild disease, 2–4 moderate, and ≥5 severe.

Admit if:

• Moderate or severe croup, or impending respiratory failure.
• RR >60.
• 'Toxic' appearance.

Milder illness may require admission if there are other factors, e.g. poor oral intake (<50–75% usual volume or no wet nappy for 12 hours), a suboptimal social situation, or parental concern.

## References

https://cks.nice.org.uk/croup
BMJ Best Practice (2017) *Croup*. https://bestpractice.bmj.com/topics/en-gb/681

## 2.5 **Sexual Health**

### Instructions for Candidate

Please take a history and discuss the management with this patient who has presented to the ED with a personal problem.

### Mark Scheme Breakdown

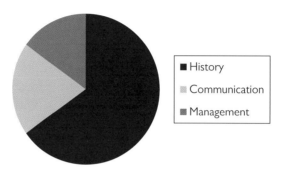

- ■ History
- ▦ Communication
- ■ Management

**Figure 2.5.1** Sexual health mark scheme breakdown.

### Instructions for Actor

You are a 23-year-old male who has presented to the ED. You have noticed some yellow discharge from the tip of your penis and it is also painful to urinate. You are worried you have a sexually transmitted infection (STI). You have not noticed any lumps or ulcers and you feel well in yourself. You have had multiple female partners (no male partners or sex workers) and do not routinely use barrier contraception. Your most recent sexual encounter was with a female acquaintance three days ago. You have previously been treated for Chlamydia. You are fit and well, take no regular medications, and have no allergies. You binge-drink at weekends but do not use any illicit drugs.

### Instructions for Examiner

Observation only.

### Equipment Required

None.

# Mark Scheme

| | |
|---|---|
| Introduces self to the patient | |
| Checks level of comfort/need for analgesia. Ensures an appropriate environment | |
| Asks an open question to elicit the presenting complaint | |
| Specifically enquires about symptoms: | |
| • Penile discharge | |
| • Pain | |
| • Dysuria | |
| • Ulcers, skin changes | |
| • Testicular lumps | |
| • Anal/perianal symptoms | |
| • Associated symptoms: dry/sore eyes, abdominal pain, joint pain | |
| • Systemic symptoms | |
| Enquires about circumstances surrounding presentation: | |
| • With whom was the sexual contact? Male/female/sex worker/from high-risk country/intravenous drug user (IVDU) | |
| • Was barrier contraception used? | |
| • Oral/vaginal/anal—received/given | |
| Enquires about sexual history: | |
| • Other sexual partners (number and type in last six months, type of sex, and contraception used) | |
| • Previous diagnosis/treatment of STIs | |
| • Previous sexual health screen or test for human immunodeficiency virus (HIV) and hepatitis | |
| Past medical history | |
| Drug history, including hepatitis B vaccination and allergies | |
| Social history, including drugs and alcohol and travel to high-risk countries | |
| Asks if there are specific concerns | |
| Explains possibility of infection | |
| Advises: | |

| | |
|---|---|
| • Sexual health screen for STI and blood-borne viruses via genitourinary (GU) clinic and offers clear instructions on how to access this | |
| • Abstinence until diagnosed and treatment complete | |
| • Use of condoms thereafter | |
| Discusses contact tracing if STI confirmed | |
| Approaches patient in non-judgemental manner | |

Total    /**27**

## Learning Points

It is important to have a non-judgemental manner and to be able to ask relevant personal questions in a sensitive way. Explain that the answers may help you make the correct diagnosis. The more you practise asking these questions without blushing, the more professional and standard procedure it will seem to the patient.

For female patients, remember to ask about contraception and menstrual history, as well as recent cervical cytology testing and pregnancy. Confirm last menstrual period (LMP) dates and consider emergency contraception (EC) if necessary.

## References

https://www.bashhguidelines.org/media/1078/sexual-history-taking-guideline-2013-2.pdf
https://www.bashh.org/guidelines

## 2.6  Lost Condom

### Instructions for Candidate

A 19-year-old female has presented to the ED concerned that a condom used in a recent sexual encounter may still be inside her vagina. Please take a history and discuss the management.

### Mark Scheme Breakdown

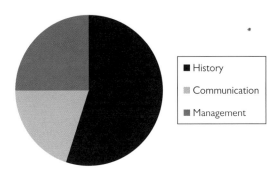

**Figure 2.6.1** Lost condom mark scheme breakdown.

### Instructions for Actor

You are a 19-year-old female who has presented to the ED, concerned that a condom used in a recent sexual encounter has been lost. You had vaginal sex last night and were unable to find the used condom afterwards. You have had a regular partner for the last six months and no other partners. You routinely use condoms and are also on the combined oral contraceptive pill (COCP). However, you have had a stressful week with exams and you have missed taking your pill three times this week. You are embarrassed about missing your pills so will only offer this information if asked. You are at university and do not wish to get pregnant. You are worried you have an STI because although your current partner is your first sexual partner, you know he has had several sexual partners before you. However, pregnancy is your biggest fear. You are fit and well, take no regular medications, and have no allergies. You drink alcohol socially on weekends but do not use illicit drugs.

### Instructions for Examiner

Observation only.

### Equipment Required

None.

## Mark Scheme

| | |
|---|---|
| Introduces self to patient | |
| Ensures privacy and checks patient comfort/offers analgesia | |
| Asks an open question to elicit presenting complaint | |
| Specifically enquires about timing of sexual intercourse in relation to presentation | |
| Asks about possible infective symptoms: | |
| • Discharge (offensive, colour, amount) | |
| • Bleeding | |
| • Vaginal pain or discomfort/dyspareunia | |
| • Abdominal pain | |
| • Urinary symptoms | |
| • Fever | |
| Enquires if she is using other forms of contraception | |
| Enquires about concordance of taking her COCP and LMP, and elicits the need for EC | |
| Enquires about her menstrual history | |
| Enquires about sexual history, particularly with reference to previous STI | |
| Confirms no other sexual partners and risk status of current partner | |
| Past medical history | |
| Drug history and allergies | |
| Social history, including drugs and alcohol | |
| Elicits ideas, concerns, and expectations | |
| Consents and offers chaperone for examination ± retrieval of condom | |
| Discusses: | |
| • EC; offers and explains how to use EC; takes a further pregnancy test if period late | |
| • Possibility of STI and suggests STI screen | |
| • Signposting how to self-refer to the GU clinic | |
| • Performing a pregnancy test | |

| | |
|---|---|
| Advises seeing her GP/family planning clinic to discuss future contraception options | |
| Approaches the patient in a non-judgemental manner | |
| Summarises the consultation and answers any further questions | |

Total     /**27**

# Learning Points

*Rules for Missed Contraceptive Pills*

*Combined Oral Contraceptive Pill*

- If one pill is missed anywhere in the pack, there is no need for EC.
- If two or more pills are missed, advise the patient to use extra contraception (e.g. condoms) for the next seven days.
- If two or more pills were missed in the first week of the pack and there has been unprotected sexual intercourse (UPSI) in the previous seven days, advise the patient to take EC.

*Progesterone-Only Pill*

- If a pill is missed or >3 hours late (or 12 hours if taking a desogestrel progesterone-only pill), extra contraception is required for the next two days. If there is UPSI during this time, advise the patient to take EC.

*Emergency Contraception Following UPSI or Contraception Failure*

- **Copper intrauterine device (IUD)**: the most effective method of EC. Inhibits fertilisation. Can be fitted up to five days after UPSI or ovulation, whichever is longer. Not known to be affected by high body mass index (BMI) or other drugs. Provides immediate ongoing contraception.
- **Oral EC**: delays ovulation. Not effective after ovulation has taken place.
  - *Ulipristal acetate (ellaOne®)*: oral EC licensed up to 120 hours after UPSI. Not recommended in women with severe asthma managed with steroids, those with hepatic impairment, or those taking an enzyme inducer.
  - *Levonorgestrel (Levonelle®)*: oral EC licensed up to 72 hours after UPSI. Effectiveness reduced if BMI >26 kg/m² or weight >70 kg, so consider double dose in these patients.

# References

https://www.nhs.uk/conditions/contraception/miss-combined-pill/
https://www.nhs.uk/conditions/contraception/miss-progestogen-only-pill/
https://www.fsrh.org/standards-and-guidance/documents/
    ceu-clinical-guidance-emergency-contraception-march-2017/
https://www.fpa.org.uk/sites/default/files/pdf/FPA%20Guide%20to%20emergency%20contraception%20
    1009.pdf

## 2.7 Febrile Convulsion

### Instructions for Candidate

Please take a history and discuss the management with the parent of a child who has presented to the ED after a seizure. At triage the child is alert, febrile, and tachycardic, but stable.

### Mark Scheme Breakdown

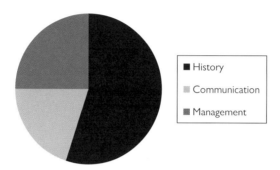

**Figure 2.7.1** Febrile convulsion mark scheme breakdown.

### Instructions for Actor

You are the parent of 18-month-old Archie who has been unwell for two days with a runny nose and a cough. You think that his throat is sore, as he has sounded a bit hoarse today. He has been off his food today but drinking well. He has had no diarrhoea or vomiting. You have not noticed any rashes. Just before bedtime, he had a seizure that you think lasted about a minute. He looked vacant; then his arms and legs started shaking and his lips looked blue. When the seizure stopped, you noticed that he felt hot to touch. He came around quickly and was crying for the next 15 minutes. He has been subdued since then. You called an ambulance and the paramedics told you he had a fever and that was why he fitted. He was born at 35 weeks but did not spend much time in hospital and has not had any issues since. He is developing well and meeting milestones as expected. He has missed his last set of immunisations as you have recently moved and have not yet registered with a GP. His eight-year-old brother has epilepsy and you are worried this is the start of Archie having epilepsy.

### Instructions for Examiner

Observation only.

### Equipment Required

None.

# Mark Scheme

| | |
|---|---|
| Introduces self and checks parent's and child's identity | |
| Confirms the triage observations are up-to-date and the child is comfortable | |
| Asks an open question to elicit the presenting complaint | |
| Elicits details regarding the seizure: | |
| • Events preceding the seizure | |
| • Description of the seizure | |
| • Timing of the seizure | |
| • Trauma/head injury before or during the seizure | |
| Elicits details regarding the resolution of the seizure: | |
| • Speed of recovery | |
| • Drowsiness | |
| • Weakness. Are all limbs moving symmetrically? | |
| • Responding normally to parents? | |
| Symptoms of illness (cough, coryza, diarrhoea and vomiting, fever, rash, oral intake, activity levels) | |
| Past medical history | |
| Pregnancy and birth history | |
| Drug history (including immunisations and recent use of antibiotics) and allergies | |
| Family history | |
| Social history, including drugs, alcohol, childcare settings, and social care input | |
| Asks if there are specific concerns | |
| Explains the diagnosis of febrile convulsion: | |
| • What a febrile convulsion is | |
| • Discusses the prognosis and chance of recurrence | |
| • Addresses the parent's concern regarding epilepsy | |
| • Acknowledges that this was a frightening experience for the family | |
| Explains the need to examine the child and conduct bedside tests (BM, urinalysis) | |
| Advises: | |

| | |
|---|---|
| • Antipyretics for symptomatic relief | |
| • How to manage any future seizure: recovery position, call 999 if duration is >5 minutes or if concerned | |
| • Registering with the GP to arrange catch-up immunisations | |
| Provides a written advice and information leaflet | |
| Discharges with advice to return if further seizures or concerns regarding child's symptoms | |

Total    /**28**

# Learning Points

*Useful Information to Give to Parents*

Febrile convulsions are associated with fever and are common in children between six months and five years of age. They occur in about 3% of children. They are generally benign and children make a complete recovery. One in three children will have a recurrence during a subsequent infection. This is not an epileptic seizure. There is a slightly increased risk of epilepsy, compared to the general population: 1/50 vs 1/100. It is recommended to follow the usual immunisation schedule, even if a febrile convulsion occurred after a vaccination.

*Consider Admission If*

- <18 months.
- Meningism.
- Complex or prolonged.
- Unexplained fever and no source of infection.
- Unwell.
- Recent antibiotics.
- Parental anxiety or poor social situation.

# References

https://cks.nice.org.uk/febrile-seizure
BMJ Best Practice (2019) *Febrile seizure.* https://bestpractice.bmj.com/topics/en-gb/566

## 2.8 **Sore Throat**

### Instructions for Candidate

Your new Senior House Officer (SHO) asks you to review this three-and-a-half-year-old child with a sore throat and to discuss antibiotic options with his parent. She tells you that his tonsils are inflamed, but with no exudate or pus present; his temperature is normal, and his RR, $O_2$ saturations, pulse, and blood pressure (BP) are within normal range for his age. His tympanic membranes appear normal; his chest is clear on auscultation, with normal heart sounds, and he has no evidence of a rash.

Please take a history and discuss the management with the parent.

### Mark Scheme Breakdown

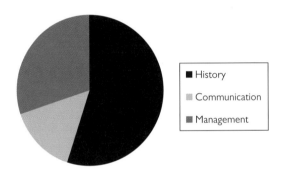

**Figure 2.8.1** Sore throat mark scheme breakdown.

### Instructions for Actor

You are the parent of George who is three-and-a-half years old. He has been unwell for two days with a fever, a sore throat and a mild cough. He has had a runny nose and has not been as hungry or playful as normal. He spent all day on the sofa, which is not like him. You have given him paracetamol three times today already, which you think has helped make him feel better. His older brother William had his tonsils removed last summer for recurrent tonsillitis and you are worried that George will need his removing soon too. You also think he needs antibiotics for his tonsillitis. George is allergic to penicillin.

### Instructions for Examiner

Observation only.

### Equipment Required

None.

## Mark Scheme

| | |
|---|---|
| Introduces self to the parent and patient | |
| Checks level of comfort/need for analgesia | |
| Asks an open question to elicit presenting complaint | |
| Specifically enquires about symptoms: | |
| • Fever in the last 24 hours | |
| • Timing of illness | |
| • Cough | |
| • Coryzal symptoms | |
| • Diarrhoea and vomiting | |
| • Rash | |
| • Eating and drinking and urinary output | |
| • Alertness and activity levels | |
| Past medical history | |
| Family history | |
| Drug history, allergies, and immunisations | |
| Social history | |
| Asks if there are specific concerns or expectations | |
| Calculates FeverPAIN = 3 | |
| Explains the diagnosis | |
| Explains antibiotics are not immediately indicated | |
| Discusses delayed or backup antibiotic prescription if no improvement in 3–5 days or if symptoms worsen | |
| Advises to return if patient's symptoms worsen rapidly or patient becomes very unwell | |
| Advises to return for review in seven days if no better | |
| Offers advice on self-care (drinking plenty of fluids, taking regular paracetamol) | |
| Appropriately negotiates management with the parent and manages their concerns | |

Total    /**24**

# Learning Points

The FeverPAIN and Centor criteria are clinical scoring tools described in the NICE guidelines that help identify patients in whom streptococcal infection is a likely cause of their sore throat and thus who are more likely to benefit from antibiotics. Often the most difficult part of the consultation is managing expectations and explaining to parents why antibiotics may or may not be needed. For a history and communication station, you must explore and discuss parental concerns and expectations.

### Explanation of No Antibiotic Approach to Parents

Most are viral illnesses and will be self-limiting; 85% of patients with tonsillitis will recover in seven days, and 80% with acute otitis media will recover in three days.

There is a risk–benefit consideration for antibiotics. Risks include reaction, side effects, allergy, resistance, and distress to the child taking them.

### Antibiotic Guidelines for Tonsillitis

Antibiotics are recommended if:

- Systemically unwell.
- Complications such as quinsy/cellulitis.
- Significant comorbidities, including premature babies.
- Three or more of the Centor criteria.

Phenoxymethylpenicillin (penicillin V) is the first-choice antibiotic. If you decide not to prescribe antibiotics, suggest a review at seven days if symptoms are not resolving.

# References

https://www.nice.org.uk/guidance/ng84/resources/visual-summary-pdf-4723226606
https://cks.nice.org.uk/sore-throat-acute#!topicSummary

## 2.9  Pneumothorax

### Instructions for Candidate

Please take a history and discuss the management with this patient who has presented to the ED.

### Mark Scheme Breakdown

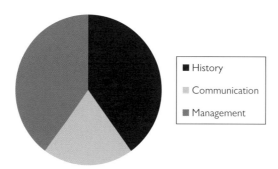

**Figure 2.9.1**  Pneumothorax mark scheme breakdown.

### Instructions for Actor

You are a 23-year-old man presenting to the ED with sudden-onset chest pain. It is sharp and worse on deep inspiration, and you feel breathless. You have no cough or fever and otherwise feel well. You have never had anything like this before. You are normally fit and healthy, with no previous medical history and no regular medications. You have no allergies. You are a non-smoker. You drink alcohol mostly at weekends. You are a keen diver and are due to fly to Egypt for a diving holiday in four weeks.

### Instructions for Examiner

Provide the candidate with an image of the chest X-ray (CXR) (Fig. 2.9.2).

### Equipment Required

CXR of pneumothorax (Fig. 2.9.2).

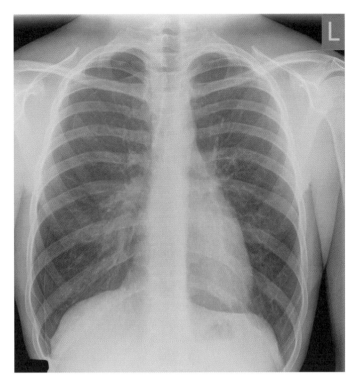

**Figure 2.9.2** Chest X-ray.

## Mark Scheme

| | |
|---|---|
| Introduces self to the patient | |
| Checks level of comfort/need for analgesia | |
| Asks an open question to elicit the presenting complaint | |
| Specifically enquires about symptoms: | |
| • Pain history (site, onset, character, radiation, exacerbating and relieving factors) | |
| • Breathlessness at rest and on exertion | |
| • Cough/productive | |
| • Systemic symptoms | |

| | |
|---|---|
| Past medical history | |
| Drug history and allergies | |
| Family history | |
| Social history, including smoking, drugs, and alcohol | |
| Asks if there are specific concerns | |
| Correctly interprets the chest radiograph | |
| Explains the diagnosis of primary spontaneous pneumothorax | |
| Explains the management: | |
| • Analgesia | |
| • No need for aspiration of pneumothorax as <2 cm | |
| • May be discharged with follow-up/safety net advice | |
| Recommends that diving must be avoided | |
| Explains that flying should be avoided for at least one week following complete radiological resolution of pneumothorax | |
| Acknowledges the impact of the diagnosis on the patient's holiday plans | |
| Offers written advice about the diagnosis and management | |
| Offers safety net advice and ensures follow-up with the respiratory team | |

Total    /**22**

# Learning Points

Fig. 2.9.3 summarises the British Thoracic Society (BTS) guidelines on the management of a spontaneous pneumothorax.

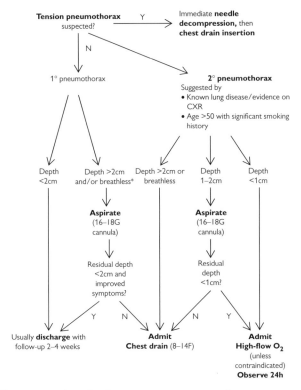

**Figure 2.9.3** BTS treatment algorithm for spontaneous pneumothorax.

From Fig 37.1 Oxford Handbook of Respiratory Medicine 3 Edn by Stephen Chapman, Grace Robinson, John Stradling, Sophie West, and John Wrightson. Oxford University Press. ISBN 9780198703860.

The BTS advises avoiding diving permanently, unless the patient has normal lung function tests and a normal CT chest following bilateral surgical pleurectomy (or other definitive prevention strategies).

Flying is not recommended until full resolution of the pneumothorax on chest radiograph. Although medical recommendation is often to avoid flying for six weeks, the UK Civil Aviation Authority states that it should be safe to travel after two weeks. According to the BTS, the risk of recurrence of pneumothorax only significantly falls after one year, so some patients may prefer to avoid air travel for that period.

# References

https://thorax.bmj.com/content/thoraxjnl/65/Suppl_2/ii18.full.pdf

https://thorax.bmj.com/content/thoraxjnl/57/4/289.full.pdf

https://www.caa.co.uk/Passengers/Before-you-fly/Am-I-fit-to-fly/Guidance-for-health-professionals/
    Respiratory-disease/

## 2.10 **Breathlessness**

### Instructions for Candidate

Please take a history and discuss the management with this patient who has presented with breathlessness. A brief examination has revealed a pulse of 95 bpm and there are no signs of haemodynamic instability.

### Mark Scheme Breakdown

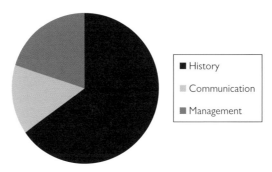

■ History

░ Communication

■ Management

**Figure 2.10.1** Breathlessness mark scheme breakdown.

### Instructions for Actor

You are a 39-year-old woman and have noticed that you have been increasingly breathless over the past two days, despite increasing your inhalers. You do not feel wheezy as you normally would with an asthma exacerbation. You have had a mild cough that is not productive and you have not coughed up any blood. You have had some uncomfortable chest pain on the right side of your chest that is worse on inspiration. You have not had a fever or any coryzal symptoms. You had ankle stabilisation surgery six weeks ago and were immobile for three days before starting to move around on crutches. You are moving around a lot more now but are not back to running yet. You have no calf swelling or pain. You do not think you are pregnant as you take a combined oral contraceptive pill. You have asthma that is treated with Clenil Modulite® twice daily (BD) and salbutamol as needed (PRN). You have never had a deep vein thrombosis (DVT) or pulmonary embolism (PE) in the past. You work in an office. You are teetotal but smoke ten cigarettes a day.

### Instructions for Examiner

Observation only.

### Equipment Required

None.

# Mark Scheme

| | |
|---|---|
| Introduces self to the patient | |
| Checks patient comfort/need for analgesia | |
| Asks an open question regarding the reason for the attendance | |
| Checks symptoms: | |
| • Shortness of breath (SOB): onset, exercise tolerance, exacerbating and relieving factors | |
| • Chest pain | |
| • Cough, haemoptysis | |
| • Fever | |
| • Symptoms of DVT | |
| • Syncope/collapse | |
| Asks about immobilisation and surgery within the last six weeks | |
| Past medical history, including specifically: | |
| • Previous DVT/PE | |
| • Previous cancer diagnosis | |
| • Obstetric history | |
| Drug history and allergies | |
| Social history | |
| Explains what a PE is | |
| Uses two-level PE Wells score to estimate the clinical probability of PE Score of 4 or less (PE unlikely) | |
| Suggests quantitative D-dimer test | |
| Explains what the next steps are if the test is positive: CT pulmonary angiography (CTPA), anticoagulation | |
| Addresses any specific concerns or questions | |

Total    /**21**

# Learning Points

Patients with suspected PE should be admitted if there are signs of haemodynamic instability or if they are pregnant or given birth within the past six weeks. Otherwise, NICE recommends using the **two-level PE Wells score** to estimate the clinical probability of PE.

PE in pregnancy and puerperium: the D-dimer test should not be performed to investigate acute venous thromboembolism (VTE) in pregnancy. In women who also have signs and symptoms of a DVT, compression ultrasonography should be performed. If DVT is confirmed, no further investigation is necessary and the patient should be treated for VTE.

NICE recommendation is to consider using the Pulmonary Embolism Rule-out Criteria (PERC) rule[*] (in non-pregnant patients) if clinical suspicion of PE is low. If all of the eight criteria are present in a patient with a low pre-test probability of PE, then PE can be ruled out clinically. The criteria are:

- Age <50 years.
- Pulse <100 bpm.
- Oxygen saturation of arterial blood ($SaO_2$) ≥95%.
- No haemoptysis.
- No oestrogen use.
- No surgery/trauma requiring hospitalisation within four weeks.
- No prior VTE.
- No unilateral leg swelling.

# References

https://www.nice.org.uk/guidance/ng158
https://www.rcog.org.uk/globalassets/documents/guidelines/gtg-37b.pdf

[*] Adapted from Table 23.2 in *The Saint-Chopra Guide to Inpatient Medicine* 4th Edition. Edited by Sanjay Saint and Vineet Chopra. Published Oxford University Press. ISBN 9780190862800.

## 2.11 **Post-partum Haemorrhage**

### Instructions for Candidate

Please take a history and discuss the management with this patient who has presented to the ED with vaginal bleeding. She has recently had a baby and is unsure if this is normal, but she is worried enough to come to the ED. Once you have discussed your management plan with the patient, the examiner will ask you two questions.

### Mark Scheme Breakdown

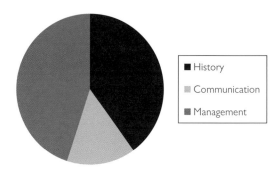

**Figure 2.11.1** Post-partum haemorrhage mark scheme breakdown.

### Instructions for Actor

You are a 35-year-old lady. You gave birth to your third child two days ago (spontaneous vaginal delivery) but have come to the ED as you are experiencing heavy blood loss and abdominal pain. You have noticed an offensive discharge per vaginum (PV), as well as the bleeding, and you feel generally unwell and light-headed. You have used two packs of maternity pads since your baby was born and are passing clots in the toilet pan. You are worried because you never felt this way with your other children. The pregnancy and birth were uncomplicated. The baby is doing well and is being mix-fed with breast milk and formula, so that your partner can help out. Your medical history includes migraines and fibromyalgia. You take paracetamol and ibuprofen when needed, but today it has not provided any relief. You have no allergies. You do not smoke and have not drunk alcohol since you became pregnant.

### Instructions for Examiner

Once the candidate has explained the management plan to the patient, please ask the following questions:

What is your differential diagnosis?

If the patient had presented 24 hours ago, how would your differential diagnosis and
   management alter?

# Equipment Required

None.

# Mark Scheme

| | |
|---|---|
| Introduces self to the patient | |
| Checks level of comfort/need for analgesia | |
| Asks an open question to elicit the presenting complaint | |
| Specifically enquires about symptoms: | |
| • Blood loss: amount, clots, number of pads used | |
| • Vaginal discharge: foul-smelling or offensive, colour | |
| • Abdominal pain | |
| • Systemic symptoms: fever/light-headedness/collapse/syncope | |
| Obstetric history | |
| Past medical history | |
| Drug history and allergies | |
| Family history | |
| Social history, including drugs and alcohol | |
| Asks if there are specific concerns | |
| Explains the need to examine the patient (abdominal, PV, and speculum) and investigate for causes of post-partum haemorrhage (PPH), e.g. retained tissue endometritis | |
| Explains the management: | |
| • To review observation chart | |
| • Analgesia | |
| • IV access and bloods: full blood count (FBC), C-reactive protein (CRP), group and save, coagulation screen | |
| • Ultrasound | |
| • Referral to obstetric team | |
| • Antibiotics (PO or IV, depending on clinical findings) | |
| • To admit if patient unwell or haemodynamically unstable | |

| | |
|---|---|
| Reassures the patient that the baby can stay with mum and breastfeeding can continue | |
| Asks if there are any further questions | |
| Answers the examiner's question regarding differential diagnosis | |
| Answers the examiner's question regarding primary PPH | |

Total    **/25**

## Learning Points

Primary PPH is bleeding within 24 hours of delivery. The four common causes are problems with uterine tone, retained tissue, tears or trauma, and coagulation.

Secondary PPH is bleeding 24 hours to 12 weeks post-partum. Consider causes such as infection or retained tissue. Management depends somewhat on the clinical presentation and can range from oral antibiotics to activation of the massive transfusion protocol in the haemodynamically unstable patient.

Remember to have a holistic approach. Aim to keep mum and baby together and facilitate breast-feeding to continue.

## Reference

https://www.rcog.org.uk/en/guidelines-research-services/guidelines/gtg52/

## 2.12 **Pre-eclampsia**

### Instructions for Candidate

Please take a history and discuss the management with this patient who presented with headache and feeling generally unwell. She is currently 32 weeks into her pregnancy. She has had a long wait to be seen and is quite keen to get home so she can sleep. Her observation chart shows she is hypertensive. Urine tests confirm pregnancy and reveal proteinuria +++.

### Mark Scheme Breakdown

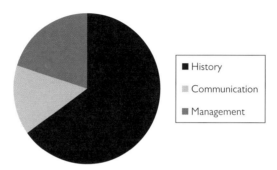

**Figure 2.12.1** Pre-eclampsia mark scheme breakdown.

### Instructions for Actor

You are a 36-year-old lady. You are 32 weeks into your fourth pregnancy. You have presented because you have a headache and heartburn that will not budge. You have not noticed any changes to your vision, and you do not think you have neurological symptoms. You feel slightly puffy, but you had this with previous pregnancies and think this is normal. You do not have any medical conditions, but you tend to avoid doctors anyway as you do not trust them. You have not fully engaged with antenatal care and have missed some recent appointments as you are worried that social services will try to take this baby away, as they did with your other children. You are scared and do not feel well, but you are keen to get some pain relief and then go home as soon as possible. You do not really understand why the high blood pressure is a problem for you or the baby. If the risks of pre-eclampsia are not properly explained to you, you will try to self-discharge.

### Instructions for Examiner

Observation only.

### Equipment Required

None.

# Mark Scheme

| | |
|---|---|
| Introduces self to the patient | |
| Checks level of comfort/need for analgesia | |
| Asks an open question to elicit the presenting complaint | |
| Specifically enquires about symptoms: | |
| • Headache: site, onset, character, radiation, associated symptoms, timing, exacerbating factors, and severity | |
| • Oedema | |
| • Abdominal pain | |
| • Visual disturbance | |
| • Feeling unwell | |
| Specifically enquires about pre-eclampsia risk factors: | |
| • Previous hypertension (previous pregnancy or pre-pregnancy) | |
| • Kidney disease, diabetes, or condition affecting the immune system | |
| • First pregnancy | |
| • Multiple pregnancy | |
| • Last pregnancy >10 years ago | |
| • Age >40 years | |
| • BMI of 35 or more | |
| • Family history of pre-eclampsia | |
| Obstetric history | |
| Past medical history | |
| Family history | |
| Drug history and allergies | |
| Social history | |
| Asks if there are specific concerns | |
| Explains what pre-eclampsia is | |
| Explains that the patient has signs of severe pre-eclampsia | |
| Sensitively explains that pre-eclampsia can cause harm to the patient and the baby | |

| Management: | |
| --- | --- |
| • Investigations to include FBC, liver function tests (LFTs), renal function, and clotting after securing IV access | |
| • Urgent obstetric referral for review and admission | |
| • BP control, e.g. labetalol | |
| • Magnesium sulphate 4 g IV | |
| Reassures the patient she will be closely monitored until it is safe to deliver the baby | |

Total    /**30**

# Learning Points

Pre-eclampsia is a multi-organ disorder specific to pregnancy, the main features of which are hypertension, proteinuria, and oedema occurring after 20 weeks' gestation. Pre-eclampsia is usually diagnosed in antenatal clinics but can also be picked up in the ED—either because of concerning symptoms or as incidental findings during investigations for other conditions.

# References

https://www.nice.org.uk/guidance/ng133/resources/
     hypertension-in-pregnancy-diagnosis-and-management-pdf-66141717671365
https://www.rcog.org.uk/globalassets/documents/patients/patient-information-leaflets/pregnancy/pi-pre-
     eclampsia.pdf
Munro PT. Management of eclampsia in the accident and emergency department. *Emergency Medicine Journal*
     2000;**17**:7–11. https://emj.bmj.com/content/17/1/7

## 2.13 **Needlestick Injury**

### Instructions for Candidate

Please take a history and discuss the management with this patient who presented with a needlestick injury. He is a dental student who was administering a local anaesthetic injection when he accidentally injured himself. His supervisor advised him to come to the ED to get checked out.

### Mark Scheme Breakdown

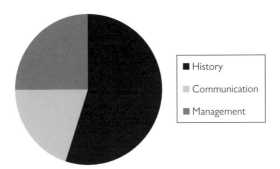

**Figure 2.13.1** Needlestick injury mark scheme breakdown.

### Instructions for Actor

You are a 23-year-old dental student in your first clinical year. You were administering a local anaesthetic injection into a patient's mouth when you accidentally stabbed your index finger with the needle. You were wearing gloves. You washed the wound and encouraged it to bleed. You told your supervisor and the patient straight away. You have completed the risk assessment form and have it with you. The source is not known to have any blood-borne viruses (BBVs) and, on questioning, is not high risk and does not come from, or live in, an area of high HIV prevalence. However, you remain incredibly worried about BBVs and are worried your career will be over unless you take immediate post-exposure prophylaxis (PEP). You are fit and healthy, with no medical problems, and you take no regular medications. You are up-to-date with occupational immunisations.

### Instructions for Examiner

Observation only.

### Equipment Required

None.

## Mark Scheme

| | |
|---|---|
| Introduces self to the patient | |
| Checks level of comfort/need for analgesia | |
| Asks an open question to elicit the presenting complaint | |
| Specifically enquires about circumstances: | |
| • Timing | |
| • Gloves | |
| • First aid administered (washed, encouraged to bleed) | |
| • Any blood in the mouth/on the needle | |
| • Depth of wound | |
| • Injected | |
| • Any broken skin | |
| Enquires about risk assessment form: | |
| • Donor factors | |
| • Needle type | |
| • Has blood been taken from donor for testing of BBVs (with consent)? | |
| Enquires about the recipient's immunisation history, including hepatitis antibody test for response | |
| Past medical history, including previous screen for HIV and hepatitis | |
| Family history | |
| Drug history and allergies | |
| Social history | |
| Asks if there are specific concerns | |
| Explains the relative risks of BBVs | |
| Explains PEP is not usually indicated in this case (no high-risk factors for HIV in source) | |
| Recognises that the patient is risk-averse and discusses the risks and benefits of PEP to reach a decision together | |
| Management: | |
| • Hepatitis B booster not required as up-to-date | |
| • Bloods for HIV, and hepatitis B and C | |

| | |
|---|---|
| • Serum save | |
| • Referral to occupational health department | |
| Explains the next steps: | |
| • Review by occupational health | |
| • Suggests patient discusses with supervisor for ongoing support | |
| Invites final questions and summarises discussion | |

Total    **/30**

## Learning Points

*Needlestick Risks*

If the source is positive, the risk of transmitting HIV is 0.3%, 3% for hepatitis C, and 30% for hepatitis B. The risk of HIV from a positive source with mucocutaneous exposure is <0.1%.

*Hepatitis B*

Knowing the hepatitis B vaccination status of the patient (and ideally the source as well) is useful to assess if they will need a full vaccination course, a hepatitis B booster, or even hepatitis B immunoglobulin. If there was significant exposure to a patient who is a known responder to the vaccine, a booster would be considered. If the patient is a non-responder, both immunoglobulin and a booster would be given. Chapter 18 of the *Green Book* provides useful treatment options for different scenarios.

*Post-Exposure Prophylaxis*

PEP should be offered if the donor is positive or high risk. If given in <1 hour, PEP will reduce the risk of HIV transmission by 80%. It can be given up to 72 hours from exposure, but ideally PEP is given as soon after the exposure as possible.

There is no need for PEP for exposure to saliva, stool, vomit, or urine unless visibly bloodstained. There is usually no need for PEP for needlestick injuries from discarded needles; however, hepatitis B can live for up to seven days.

## References

https://www.nhs.uk/common-health-questions/medicines/can-post-exposure-prophylaxis-pep-stop-me-getting-hiv/

BMJ Best Practice (2018) *Post-exposure HIV prophylaxis.* https://bestpractice.bmj.com/topics/en-gb/1109

https://assets.publishing.service.gov.uk/government/uploads/system/uploads/attachment_data/file/628602/Greenbook_chapter__18.pdf

https://patient.info/doctor/needlestick-injury-pro

## 2.14 **Transient Loss of Consciousness**

### Instructions for Candidate

This 48-year-old male has been brought into the ED, accompanied by his wife, following an episode of loss of consciousness. He had been to a restaurant for dinner when this happened. He feels fine now and thinks his wife is making a fuss about nothing. His observation chart shows normal vital signs. Please take a history and advise him on the best management plan.

### Mark Scheme Breakdown

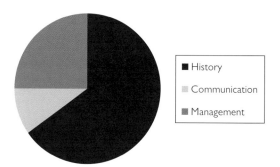

- History
- Communication
- Management

**Figure 2.14.1** TLOC mark scheme breakdown.

### Instructions for Actor

You are 48 years old. You were celebrating your fifteenth wedding anniversary with your wife at your favourite restaurant. You and your wife shared a bottle of wine with dinner. You had slightly more than half the bottle but did not feel drunk. After the meal, you were standing at the bar and felt light-headed. You had no chest pain, palpitations, or breathlessness, and no headache, aura, or weakness. Your wife saw you collapse and lose consciousness for about 20 seconds before recovery. During the event, you were incontinent of urine, which you find incredibly embarrassing. You did not bite your tongue. You did not have any limb-jerking. You recovered quickly, but an ambulance had already been called and your wife insisted on getting you checked out. You have no previous medical history. You do not take any regular medication and have no allergies. You are in a stressful job and like to relax by drinking half a bottle of wine in the evening. You do not smoke. You want to go home as soon as possible.

### Instructions for Examiner

Provide the candidate with a copy of the electrocardiogram (ECG) (Fig. 2.14.2).

# Equipment Required

ECG (Fig. 2.14.2).

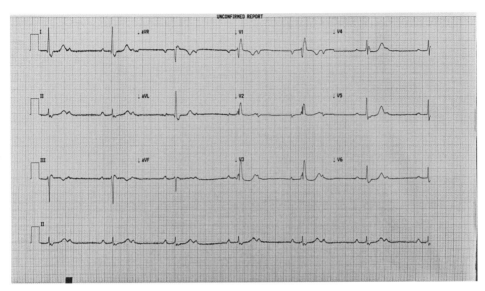

**Figure 2.14.2** ECG case 2.14.

# Mark Scheme

| | |
|---|---|
| Introduces self to the patient | |
| Checks level of comfort/need for analgesia | |
| Asks an open question to elicit the presenting complaint | |
| Specifically enquires about circumstances preceding the event: | |
| • Posture | |
| • Provoking factors, e.g. pain, urination, opening bowels, cough | |
| • Prodrome | |
| Specifically enquires about symptoms: | |
| • Cardiac symptoms: chest pain, palpitations, breathlessness, light-headedness | |
| • Neurological symptoms: headache, weakness, facial droop, visual disturbance, speech disturbance, altered sensation, aura, seizures | |
| Events during the transient loss of consciousness (TLOC) (confirms with his wife as a witness) | |

| | |
|---|---|
| • Appearance and colour during the event | |
| • Presence or absence of movements, e.g. limb-jerking | |
| • Tongue-biting or other injuries | |
| • Duration of event | |
| Events following TLOC: | |
| • Confusion | |
| • Recollection of events | |
| • Time to full recovery | |
| • Unilateral weakness | |
| Brief systems review | |
| Past medical history, including previous TLOC | |
| Family history—specifically cardiac disease/sudden cardiac death | |
| Drug history and allergies | |
| Social history, including drugs and alcohol | |
| Asks if there are specific concerns | |
| Explains the need for physical examination | |
| Explains need for initial investigations: | |
| • 12-lead ECG (correctly interprets as Mobitz type 2) | |
| • Other investigations, e.g. blood sugar, FBC, lying and standing BP | |
| Explains that the ECG is abnormal and considered a red flag for referral | |
| Advises admission to cardiology for pacemaker insertion | |
| If the patient refuses admission, arranges urgent referral and advises the patient not to drive whilst waiting for specialist assessment | |
| Summarises discussion and answers any questions the patient might have | |

Total    /**29**

## Learning Points

TLOC is a common ED presentation. It is important to gauge from the history whether it is an uncomplicated vasovagal syncope (ask about posture, provoking factors, and prodrome—the three Ps) or situational syncope (e.g. micturition, fear, etc.). These patients can be given a copy of their ECG, an advice leaflet, and follow-up with the GP if further similar episodes occur.

If it is not uncomplicated syncope, the history should elicit other causes such as orthostatic hypotension, cardiac (e.g. structural or arrhythmias) or neurally mediated syncope, or even a simple fall or epilepsy.

NICE recommends a specialist cardiovascular assessment within 24 hours for patients with red flag features, which include:

- ECG abnormality.
- Heart failure (history or signs).
- TLOC during exertion.
- Family history of sudden cardiac death or inherited cardiac condition.
- New/unexplained breathlessness.
- Heart murmur.

You must advise about driving restrictions following TLOC unless it is a simple faint. According to the Driver and Vehicle Licensing Agency (DVLA), road traffic collisions due to blackouts are two to three times more common than collisions caused by seizures.

## References

https://pathways.nice.org.uk/pathways/transient-loss-of-consciousness
https://www.gov.uk/government/publications/assessing-fitness-to-drive-a-guide-for-medical-professionals

## 2.15  Vertigo

### Instructions for Candidate

This 56-year-old gentleman presented to the ED with dizziness that he has experienced since lunch-time, after his game of tennis. Please take a history and discuss the management with the patient.

### Mark Scheme Breakdown

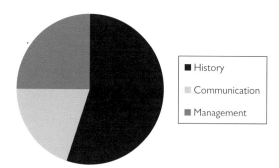

**Figure 2.15.1** Vertigo mark scheme breakdown.

### Instructions for Actor

You are a 56-year-old man who has presented to the ED to help get rid of your dizziness. You were well this morning and enjoyed a game of tennis, but after lunch, you became dizzy. If asked, you say you feel the world is spinning around you and is relatively constant. You are also struggling to walk and feel uncoordinated. You have not noticed a significant difference when you move your head. You feel slightly nauseated but have not been sick. You have no hearing loss or tinnitus. You have never had this before. You take ramipril for hypertension, which was diagnosed ten years ago. You quit smoking two years ago and drink about 21 units of alcohol per week. You have a high-pressured job and are due to drive to London to lead an important international conference tomorrow, but you are struggling with your symptoms.

### Instructions for Examiner

Observation only.

### Equipment Required

None.

# Mark Scheme

| | |
|---|---|
| Introduces self to the patient | |
| Checks level of comfort/need for analgesia | |
| Asks an open question to elicit the presenting complaint | |
| Clarifies the symptom is true vertigo, as opposed to pre-syncope, light-headedness, etc. | |
| Asks specifically about vertigo symptoms: | |
| • Timing—onset, duration, frequency | |
| • Exacerbating factors, e.g. head movement | |
| • Severity and impact on daily activities | |
| Asks about associated symptoms: | |
| • Nausea and vomiting | |
| • Hearing loss, tinnitus, ear pain or discharge | |
| • Neurological—weakness, visual disturbance, speech disturbance, headache, ataxia, aura | |
| Asks about recent head or ear trauma | |
| Past medical history | |
| Family history | |
| Drug history and allergies | |
| Social history, including drugs and alcohol | |
| Asks if there are specific concerns | |
| Explains the need for physical examination—neurological and ear, nose, and throat (ENT) | |
| Offers medication to alleviate nausea, e.g. prochlorperazine | |
| Explains the need for investigations, including CT/magnetic resonance imaging (MRI) for central causes of vertigo, e.g. stroke (concerns regarding vertigo plus poor coordination and difficulty walking) | |
| Advises urgent specialist neurological review, in line with local stroke pathways | |
| Sensitively discusses and manages the patient's expectations and concerns | |
| Advises not to drive whilst waiting for specialist assessment | |
| Summarises discussion and answers any questions the patient might have | |

Total    /**23**

## Learning Points

The challenge with a patient presenting with dizziness is to distinguish what is meant by the term, which could describe symptoms of vertigo, pre-syncope, disequilibrium, or light-headedness. The presence of nystagmus indicates that the dizziness is likely vertigo. Once it is ascertained that vertigo is the presenting symptom, it is important to take a careful history and perform a thorough examination to determine whether the vertigo is due to central (i.e. pathology of the brain, e.g. brainstem or cerebellum) or peripheral causes (usually inner ear problems affecting the labyrinth or vestibular nerve). The management of vertigo includes symptomatic relief, e.g. anti-emetics and IV fluids if vomiting is a significant feature, and subsequently depends on the suspected cause of the vertigo. If stroke is suspected, immediate management is required, in line with local stroke pathways.

## References

https://cks.nice.org.uk/vertigo
https://www.nice.org.uk/guidance/ng127/chapter/
   Recommendations-for-adults-aged-over-16#dizziness-and-vertigo-in-adults

## 2.16 Sickle Cell Crisis

### Instructions for Candidate

Please take a history and advise on the best management for this patient who has presented with acute joint pain and is requesting strong painkillers. There is no need to examine the patient.

### Mark Scheme Breakdown

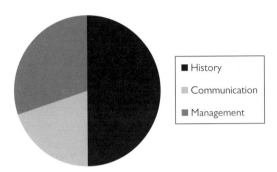

**Figure 2.16.1** Sickle cell crisis mark scheme breakdown.

### Instructions for Actor

You are a 23-year-old university student. You have presented to the ED with acute pain in multiple joints in your hands and feet, but also your right knee is painful and a bit swollen. You have not had any injuries or falls. You have tried to manage this with regular paracetamol and ibuprofen at home, but the pain is too much and you are fed up with it. You have had this before and the only thing that has helped is morphine, which is why you are here, and you are pushing to get some prescribed now. You feel defensive as you are aware this makes you look like a drug-seeker, but you have been in this situation before many times and know what works for you. An empathetic approach by the candidate will calm and reassure you. If asked, you feel worn out and tired, which happens sometimes, but you put it down to being busy with university activities. You have no chest pain or breathlessness. You normally try to eat and drink well to maintain your fitness. Yesterday you spent most of the day in bed recovering from a big night out to celebrate handing in an assignment, which perhaps meant you became a bit dehydrated. You find that cold weather also contributes to your symptoms. Your past medical history includes sickle cell disease (SCD) and you have required blood transfusions and admissions for painful crises in the past. You are keen to get this sorted as soon as possible as you hate being in pain and you are not managing it well.

### Instructions for Examiner

Observation only.

## Equipment Required

None.

## Mark Scheme

| | |
|---|---|
| Introduces self to the patient | |
| Checks level of comfort/need for analgesia | |
| Asks an open question to elicit the presenting complaint: | |
| • Asks about injuries, falls, etc. | |
| • Asks about timing: onset of pain, duration, time of day, previous episodes | |
| • Site of pain | |
| • Associated symptoms, e.g. swelling, fever, hot and red joints | |
| • Exacerbating and relieving factors | |
| • Severity | |
| • Systems review, in particular breathlessness, chest pain, tiredness, fever, and recent infection | |
| Past medical history | |
| Family history | |
| Drug history and allergies | |
| Social history, including drugs and alcohol | |
| Asks if there are specific concerns | |
| Discusses treatment during previous episodes and the planned management for current episode | |
| Explains the need for examination to rule out other causes of joint pain, but also other complications of SCD | |
| Explains the patient may require IV fluids or top-up transfusion | |
| Prescribes opiates, in addition to regular simple analgesia | |
| Advises the patient to continue oral intake to prevent dehydration | |
| Advises admission for analgesia | |
| Explains will liaise with haematology for ongoing care and support during admission and beyond | |
| Summarises the negotiated plan and invites final questions | |

Total     /**23**

## Learning Points

Painful episodes, also known as sickle cell crises, are one of the most common symptoms of SCD. They can often be managed at home with regular simple analgesia, but moderate to severe pain may require admission for opiates (consider patient-controlled analgesia if repeated boluses of strong opiates are needed). Remember adjuncts such as laxatives and anti-emetics as needed too.

For pregnant women with an acute painful episode, liaise with the obstetric team and avoid NSAIDs.

Be aware of other possible complications such as infections, osteomyelitis, splenic sequestration, aplastic crisis, acute chest syndrome, and acute stroke.

## References

https://www.nice.org.uk/guidance/cg143/resources/sickle-cell-disease-managing-acute-painful-episodes-in-hospital-pdf-35109569155525

BMJ Best Practice (2020) *Sickle cell anaemia*. https://bestpractice.bmj.com/topics/en-gb/100

## 2.17 **Chest Pain**

### Instructions for Candidate

Please take a history and advise on the best management for this patient who has presented with chest pain. He is currently haemodynamically normal and you are not required to examine him.

### Mark Scheme Breakdown

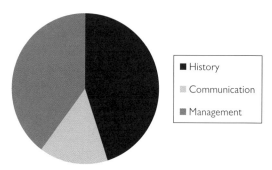

**Figure 2.17.1** Chest pain mark scheme breakdown.

### Instructions for Actor

You are a 43-year-old man who has come to the ED with chest pain. You have had panic attacks before, but this feels different. It is central chest pain and your arms feel heavy. You are not particularly breathless, but you feel sweaty and as if your heart is racing. You have not had this before. It started about an hour ago, whilst you were at the nightclub with friends. You do not volunteer it, but if asked, you disclose that you had used cocaine from a trusted source before going out. You do not believe it is the cause of your chest pain as you have used cocaine many times before without any problems. Your past medical history includes anxiety, for which you take sertraline. You smoke 20 cigarettes per day but do not drink any alcohol. Your father has angina that you believe was diagnosed in his early 60s.

### Instructions for Examiner

Provide the ECG (Fig. 2.17.2) to the candidate for review.

### Equipment Required

ECG (Fig. 2.17.2).

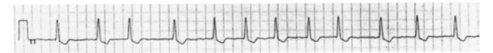

**Figure 2.17.2** ECG case 2.17.

From Fig. 16.3.1.22 Electrocardiography in Oxford Textbook Medicine (6th Edn). Edited by John Firth, Christopher Conlon.

## Mark Scheme

| | |
|---|---|
| Introduces self to the patient | |
| Checks level of comfort/need for analgesia | |
| Asks an open question to elicit the presenting complaint | |
| • Asks about the site of the pain and if it radiates | |
| • Asks about timing: onset of pain, what the patient was doing at the time, duration, and previous episodes | |
| • Associated symptoms | |
| • Exacerbating and relieving factors | |
| • Severity | |
| Past medical history | |
| Family history | |
| Drug history and allergies | |
| Social history, including drugs and alcohol | |
| Asks if there are specific concerns | |
| Explains the need for physical examination to rule out other causes of chest pain | |
| Discusses investigations, including ECG, blood tests (troponin), and CXR | |
| Reviews the ECG and recognises ischaemic changes | |
| Explains why the ECG findings are concerning | |
| Explains that cocaine use is a risk factor | |
| Explains the proposed management: | |
| • Aspirin, ticagrelor or clopidogrel—usual acute coronary syndrome (ACS) management | |

| | |
|---|---|
| • Nitrates and benzodiazepines to relieve chest pain | |
| • Admission and liaison with cardiology | |
| • Advises cessation of cocaine use and smoking, with clear signposting for support | |
| Summarises the negotiated plan and invites final questions | |

Total    /**23**

## Learning Points

Cocaine acts on alpha and beta adrenoceptors and results in increased myocardial $O_2$ demand and decreased myocardial perfusion, as well as promoting thrombus formation.

Cocaine can result in myocardial ischaemia/infarction, myocarditis, cardiomyopathy, aortic dissection, arrhythmias, and also acute strokes.

The usual management of ACS applies. In addition, in the context of cocaine use, consider the use of benzodiazepines in the management of ongoing chest pain. Remember to avoid beta-blockers in the acute management of cocaine-induced chest pain due to the risks of unopposed alpha-effect.

## References

https://pathways.nice.org.uk/pathways/chest-pain
BMJ Best Practice (2020) *Cocaine abuse*. https://bestpractice.bmj.com/topics/en-gb/199

## 2.18 **Limping Child**

### Instructions for Candidate

Please take a history from this four-year-old boy and his mother. You are not required to examine him. Vital signs are normal.

### Mark Scheme Breakdown

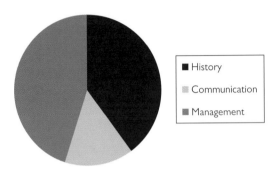

**Figure 2.18.1** Limping child mark scheme breakdown.

### Instructions for Actor

You are Harry's mother and have brought him to the ED as you are worried about his limp. You noticed it yesterday evening but thought it would just settle overnight, but it has remained throughout today. You are not aware of any trauma or injury. Harry was in nursery yesterday, but the nursery staff did not mention any injuries. The limp is on the left side—he does not seem to be putting full weight through the leg but is still mobile and he is playing happily in the waiting room. You have not noticed any bruising, rashes, or swelling. Harry was born at term, with no complications. However, he is under the care of the community paediatric team as he has global developmental delay. He can walk and run, although he was late to do so, and has speech delay, which means it is difficult to understand him. You feel he has a high pain threshold. He has recently had a fever with a cough and a runny nose, but this has resolved and he has recovered enough to go to nursery.

### Instructions for Examiner

Observation only.

### Equipment Required

None.

## Mark Scheme

| | |
|---|---|
| Introduces self to the patient and his mother | |
| Checks level of comfort/need for analgesia | |
| Asks open question to elicit the presenting complaint | |
| Establishes details of the limp: | |
| • Site of concern | |
| • Onset, timing (e.g. worse in the morning), consistency of symptoms | |
| • Associated trauma | |
| • Associated symptoms, e.g. joint swelling, redness, rash, fever | |
| • Exacerbating and relieving factors | |
| • Is he systemically well? | |
| Establishes if any preceding infections or drug exposure | |
| Past medical history, including birth history (? breech) and brief developmental history | |
| Family history, including developmental dysplasia of the hip (DDH), Perthes, rheumatological | |
| Drug history, including immunisations, and allergies | |
| Social history, including drugs and alcohol, childcare settings, social services input | |
| Enquires if mother has any specific concerns or ideas | |
| Explains need to examine the patient and observe his gait | |
| If the examination is reassuring, the likely diagnosis is transient synovitis | |
| Explains that transient synovitis is a self-limiting condition that can be managed at home | |
| Reassures there are no long-term joint problems | |
| Advises simple analgesia if needed | |
| Advises to allow patient to rest until symptoms resolve | |
| Advises review in 48 hours | |
| Explains the approach to investigations if symptoms persist at review, which would include X-ray of pelvis, including both hips, and blood tests (FBC, CRP) | |
| Offers safety net advice. To return if: | |
| • Temperature >38°C | |

| | |
|---|---|
| • Pain increases | |
| • Ongoing pain/limp after two weeks | |
| • Develops pain, swelling, or redness in any other joints | |
| Summarises the negotiated plan and invites final questions | |

Total    **/29**

## Learning Points

The differential diagnosis of an acute limp in childhood is wide, ranging from self-limiting to much more serious, e.g. septic arthritis and malignancy. A delay in treatment for septic arthritis can be devastating and cause long-lasting damage in a short period of time. Make sure this is in your differential and actively excluded. Be cautious in making a diagnosis of transient synovitis in children under three years, as it is less common in this age group. X-rays would be indicated in children with a history of trauma or bony tenderness on examination or in those older than nine years old to rule out a slipped upper femoral epiphysis. Also consider referred pain, so make sure you examine joints both above and below the hip. Sadly, non-accidental injury must always be considered. Some symptoms are red flags for serious pathology (Table 2.18.1).

**Table 2.18.1** Red flags for acute limp

| Red flags for serious pathology | Conditions to consider |
|---|---|
| Pain at night | Malignancy |
| Redness, swelling, stiffness | Infection or inflammatory joint disease |
| Weight loss, anorexia, fever, night sweats, fatigue | Malignancy, infection, inflammation |
| Unexplained rash or bruising | Haematological or inflammatory condition; non-accidental injury |
| Limp and stiffness worse in the morning | Inflammatory joint disease |
| Severe pain, anxiety, and agitation after traumatic injury | Evolving compartment syndrome |

Adapted from NICE CKS *Acute Childhood Limp* (https://cks.nice.org.uk/acute-childhood-limp).

The NICE guidelines focus on the management of limping children from a primary care perspective and state the working diagnosis would be transient synovitis if the child is 'well, afebrile, mobile but limping, and has had the symptoms for less than 48 hours'. If patients do not exhibit any of the red flags for serious pathology, the need for X-rays and bloods should be weighed against the risks of the radiation dose of an X-ray or the invasive nature of blood tests. This should be discussed with parents or legal guardians, and options, such as arranging to bring the child back in two days, with an appropriate safety net, to review the symptoms and assess the need for investigations, could be offered. Local guidelines may be available to guide management.

# References

https://cks.nice.org.uk/acute-childhood-limp#!topicSummary
BMJ Best Practice (2020) *Transient synovitis*. https://bestpractice.bmj.com/topics/en-gb/761
BMJ Best Practice (2020) *Septic arthritis*. https://bestpractice.bmj.com/topics/en-gb/486

## 2.19 **Back Pain**

### Instructions for Candidate

Please take a history and discuss with the patient the appropriate management of her back pain. You are not required to examine the patient.

### Mark Scheme Breakdown

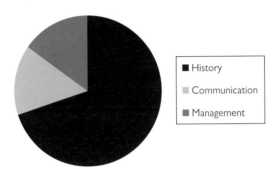

**Figure 2.19.1** Back pain mark scheme breakdown.

### Instructions for Actor

You are a 41-year-old lady who has a long history of back pain, ever since you fell off a horse in your early 20s. Over the past year, you have also experienced pain shooting down your right leg from your buttock, and your GP has diagnosed you with sciatica. You occasionally get flare-ups of worsening lower back pain, often triggered by heavy lifting or playing with the children. Today, you experienced severe pain in your lower back after you got out of the car. Your normal remedies of painkillers and heat packs have not helped, and you are feeling desperate. The co-codamol 30/500 that you use when you are having an exacerbation is not working and you are requesting something stronger. You are embarrassed about some urinary incontinence today, so you will only mention it if specifically asked. You had not realised that you had passed urine until you noticed that your clothes and the chair were wet. You are prone to constipation, but it is no worse than usual, with your bowels opening every other day. You feel otherwise fine in yourself.

Apart from back pain, you are normally healthy, only suffering from the occasional urinary tract infection (UTI). You take pregabalin, naproxen, and co-codamol. You have no allergies. You are a teaching assistant and enjoy your job. You drink alcohol socially and do not smoke. You are worried about the severity of the pain—desperate for some strong pain relief—and also the incontinence, as this has never happened before.

### Instructions for Examiner

Observation only.

## Equipment Required

None.

## Mark Scheme

| | |
|---|---|
| Introduces self to the patient | |
| Checks level of comfort/need for analgesia | |
| Asks an open question to elicit the presenting complaint | |
| Elicits further pain history: | |
| • Site, radiation | |
| • Onset, timing | |
| • Character of pain, severity | |
| • Exacerbating and relieving factors | |
| Specifically enquires about associated symptoms: | |
| • Altered sensation (e.g. saddle anaesthesia) | |
| • Bilateral sciatica | |
| • Bilateral neurological deficit of the legs | |
| • Bladder dysfunction (specifically loss of sensation when urinating and difficulty starting urination) | |
| • Bowel dysfunction | |
| • Sexual dysfunction | |
| • Fever, night sweats, weight loss | |
| Systems review to elicit further symptoms | |
| Past medical history | |
| Family history | |
| Drug history and allergies | |
| Social history, including drugs and alcohol | |
| Asks if there are specific concerns | |
| Offers a differential diagnosis | |
| Explains the need for physical examination | |
| Discusses relevant investigations and timescales | |
| Sensitively discusses and manages the patient's expectations and concerns | |

| Summarises the discussion and answers any questions the patient might have regarding onward care | |
|---|---|

Total    /25

## Learning Points

Back pain is a common ED presentation. One of the most important serious spinal pathologies to identify is cauda equina syndrome (CES), as the consequences of missing this diagnosis can be devastating for all involved. CES must be considered and excluded. NICE lists the red flags that point to possible serious spinal pain and that should form part of your history and examination.

Red flags for serious causes of spinal pain are summarised in Table 2.19.1.

**Table 2.19.1**  Red flags for serious causes of spinal pain

| Spinal fracture | Sudden onset, relieved on lying down |
|---|---|
| | History of trauma (even minor trauma if osteoporosis or steroids) |
| | Structural deformity of spine |
| | Point tenderness |
| Cancer | Age >50 years |
| | Gradual onset |
| | Unremitting pain, night pain, thoracic pain |
| | No improvement after 4–6 weeks |
| | Unexplained weight loss |
| | History of cancer |
| Infection | Fever |
| | Tuberculosis |
| | Recent UTI |
| | Diabetes |
| | IVDU |
| | HIV |
| | Immunocompromise |
| Cauda equina | Bilateral sciatica |
| | Severe/progressive bilateral neurological deficit of legs |
| | Bladder or bowel dysfunction |
| | Sexual dysfunction |
| | Saddle paraesthesiae |
| | Laxity of anal sphincter |

NB. This station could easily be turned into a communication station by omitting the red flag symptoms and explaining to the patient requesting a scan that an urgent MRI is not indicated.

Adapted from https://cks.nice.org.uk/sciatica-lumbar-radiculopathy#!diagnosisSub:1.

## Reference

https://cks.nice.org.uk/sciatica-lumbar-radiculopathy

## 2.20 **Ankle Injury**

## Instructions for Candidate

Your SHO comes to you for advice as the patient he has seen and examined is angry about his long wait to be seen and is demanding an X-ray. The SHO's examination findings did not indicate the need for an X-ray. Please review the patient, take a brief history, and discuss the management.

## Mark Scheme Breakdown

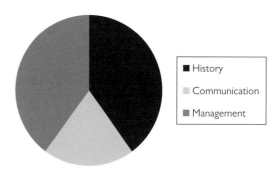

**Figure 2.20.1** Ankle injury mark scheme breakdown.

## Instructions for Actor

You are a 42-year-old man who enjoys a game of football with your colleagues after work. Today, whilst avoiding a tackle, you twisted your right ankle. If asked specifics, you demonstrate with the other ankle how your foot twisted in and the ankle inverted as you fell. It is significantly bruised and swollen. You initially tried to carry on playing but thought it might be broken as you heard a popping sound. You can put weight on it, although it is painful. Your friend brought you to the ED for an X-ray. You have waited a long time to be seen, which is making you cross, and you cannot understand why you are not being offered an X-ray. If it is offered to you, you calm down immediately. If an X-ray is not offered, you may be appeased if you receive an apology for the long wait, some reassurance about your injury, and an explanation of why an X-ray is not required.

## Instructions for Examiner

Provide the candidate with the image of the patient's ankle (Fig. 2.20.2) and the documented examination findings (Box 2.20.1).

## Equipment Required

Photo of the ankle (Fig. 2.20.2).

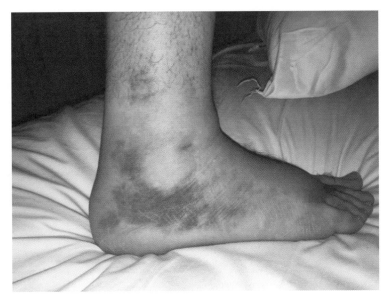

**Figure 2.20.2** Right ankle injury case 2.20.

---

**Box 2.20.1** Documentation of examination findings of right ankle injury in case 2.20

*On examination:*

*Antalgic gait, but able to weight-bear to walk down the corridor for approximately 20 steps.*

*Diffusely swollen ankle, bruising to anterolateral aspect of ankle.*

*Tender over anterior lateral malleolus and along the anterior talofibular ligament, no tenderness over posterior lateral malleolus, medial malleolus, navicular, or head of fifth metatarsal.*

*Globally reduced range of active and passive movement, especially painful on inversion.*

*Normal mid- and forefoot examination, normal knee examination.*

---

## Mark Scheme

| | |
|---|---|
| Introduces self to the patient | |
| Apologises for the long wait | |
| Checks level of comfort/need for analgesia | |
| Asks an open question to elicit the presenting complaint | |
| Elicits further pain history: | |
| • Site, radiation | |
| • Severity | |

| | |
|---|---|
| • Mechanism of injury | |
| • Exacerbating factors, e.g. ability to weight-bear, take steps | |
| Enquires about any other painful (distracting) injuries | |
| Enquires about altered sensation | |
| Past medical history | |
| Family history | |
| Drug history and allergies | |
| Social history, including drugs and alcohol | |
| Elicits patient's concerns regarding a fracture | |
| Offers to re-examine the ankle | |
| Offers a differential diagnosis | |
| Explains that ankle X-ray series are not required | |
| Explains the diagnosis of sprain and how it is best managed: | |
| • Ice | |
| • Elevation | |
| • Simple analgesia | |
| • Gentle mobilising | |
| • Offers ankle sprain advice leaflet | |
| Advises on how to access physiotherapy if pain persists | |
| Sensitively discusses and manages the patient's expectations and concerns | |
| Summarises the discussion and answers any questions the patient might have | |

Total     /**27**

# Learning Points

The Ottawa ankle and foot rules can be used to determine the need for diagnostic imaging following ankle and foot trauma. Use caution with patients with distracting injuries or who are intoxicated.

*Ottawa Ankle Rules*

An ankle X-ray is required if there is pain in the malleolar zone **and**:

- Bone tenderness at the posterior edge or tip of the lateral malleolus, **or**
- Bone tenderness at the posterior edge or tip of the medial malleolus, **or**
- An inability to bear weight both immediately and in the ED for four steps.

*Ottawa Foot Rules*

A foot X-ray is required if there is pain in the midfoot zone **and**:

- Bone tenderness at the base of the fifth metatarsal, **or**
- Bone tenderness at the navicular, **or**
- An inability to bear weight both immediately and in the ED for four steps.

# Reference

http://www.theottawarules.ca/ankle_rules

## 2.21 **Haematuria**

### Instructions for the Candidate

Please read the letter below from the patient's GP and then take a history and discuss the management. The patient has been seen in triage and catheterised already.

'*Dear colleague,*

*Please see this 69-year-old gentleman who is in urinary retention. He has been struggling to PU for the past two days and booked an urgent GP appt today to see me. I recently referred him to urology for a two-week wait appointment due to occasional mild visible haematuria and back pain. He also has a past medical history of bladder carcinoma three years ago that was treated intravesically. At the urology appointment, he was referred for an urgent CT, which he had two days ago, and I received the report this morning. It demonstrated a bladder mass that appears to be invading the detrusor muscle, with likely spinal metastases in L2 and L3. I was planning to admit directly to urology, but due to his current symptoms, I feel he probably needs admission via the ED to resolve his acute retention first. Many thanks for your help.*

*Kind regards,*

*Dr Brown*'

### Mark Scheme Breakdown

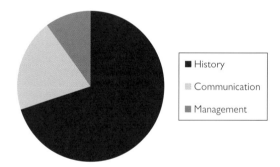

**Figure 2.21.1** Haematuria mark scheme breakdown.

### Instructions for Actor

You are 69 years old. Yesterday you started passing bright red blood. However, for the past 24 hours, it has been getting harder to pass urine and you have not managed to pass urine since the early hours of the morning. Your GP Dr Brown sent you straight to the ED with a letter. You have been seen at triage and catheterised.

You recently had an appointment with the urologists, followed by a CT scan that your GP asked for, because you had been passing pink urine four weeks ago for a few days. You are not passing urine more frequently; you have no urgency to pass urine or any pain when you pass urine. You feel you completely empty your bladder when you do go and do not have any hesitation when you start. You normally pass urine once or twice a night but have done so for the past five years. You have been getting some back pain for the past three months.

You have a medical history of hypertension, for which you take amlodipine, and you had bladder cancer three years ago but were treated and cured. You have no allergies.

If you are asked about what your understanding of the situation is, you are happy that the cancer was cured three years ago and believe that it will not come back. You are worried about the blood in your urine but think this might be from your kidneys, because you know that kidneys have something to do with high blood pressure.

## Instructions for Examiner

Observation only.

## Equipment Required

None.

## Mark Scheme

| | |
|---|---|
| Introduces self to the patient | |
| Checks level of comfort/need for analgesia | |
| Asks an open question to elicit the presenting complaint | |
| Asks about the haematuria: | |
| • When it was first noticed | |
| • Beginning or end of stream or throughout | |
| • Colour (bright red to pink tinge) | |
| • Previous history of haematuria | |
| Enquires about other urogenital symptoms: | |
| • Dysuria, frequency, urgency | |
| • Hesitancy, retention | |
| • Complete void | |
| • Nocturia—how often? | |
| • Erectile dysfunction | |
| • Testicular changes: shape, lumps | |
| • Penile changes | |

| | |
|---|---|
| Enquires about systemic symptoms and signs: | |
| • Weight loss | |
| • Back pain | |
| • Fever | |
| • High BP | |
| • Joint pains or rashes | |
| • Oedema or swelling, especially around the eyes | |
| • Pharyngitis or skin infections | |
| Enquires about recent urological interventions | |
| Enquires about recent vigorous physical activity | |
| Past medical history | |
| Family history | |
| Drug history and allergies | |
| Social history, including drugs and alcohol, travel history, and occupational history (including industrial chemical exposure) | |
| Asks if there are specific concerns | |
| Checks understanding of why the CT scan was performed and checks he knows what the CT shows | |
| Sensitively explains the diagnosis from the CT report | |
| Advises regarding the need for further urological input, as well as oncology | |
| Suggests need for up-to-date bloods: FBC, urea and electrolytes (U&E), LFTs | |
| Offers information on how to look after his catheter | |
| Sensitively discusses and manages the patient's expectations and concerns | |
| Summarises the discussion and answers any questions the patient might have | |

Total    /**35**

## Learning Points

There are many causes of haematuria and a surgical sieve is a useful way to differentiate and ensure you are asking the relevant questions in your history. Consider causes such as malignancy, infection, trauma, medical (e.g. glomerulonephritides), haematological, gynaecological, iatrogenic, and pseudohaematuria (i.e. foods or medicines that discolour the urine).

When presented with the results of investigations the patient has already had, it is good practice to check their understanding before proceeding with the consultation. That way, you ensure you can deliver information regarding diagnosis and management in a sensitive way, maintaining a good and trusting relationship with the patient.

# References

https://cks.nice.org.uk/urological-cancers-recognition-and-referral#!topicSummary
BMJ Best Practice (2020) *Assessment of visible haematuria*. https://bestpractice.bmj.com/topics/en-gb/316
https://www.macmillan.org.uk/_images/ten-tips-haematuria_tcm9-300202.pdf

## 2.22 **Abdominal Pain**

### Instructions for Candidate

Please take a history and discuss the management.

### Mark Scheme Breakdown

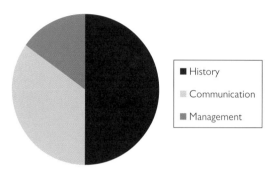

**Figure 2.22.1** Abdominal pain mark scheme breakdown.

### Instructions for Actor

*Julian*

You are Julian and you are 12 years old. You had an episode of pain this morning. Your mother sent you to school this morning as it got better quite quickly, and she thought it might be constipation again. You had a big drink and an old packet of Fybogel® before school. However, you were sent home as your pain worsened suddenly and you started to feel sick. Your mother brought you straight to the ED. You have a really sore tummy and feel sick. You have vomited twice on the way over and once in the ED. You are otherwise well with no significant medical history. If asked directly, you admit you have a very painful left testicle but are embarrassed about it, especially because it is swollen. You are scared about what is happening to you.

*Mother*

You brought your son to the ED from school as he was crying in pain, which is unusual for him. He had a brief episode of pain earlier on, but it seemed to settle a few minutes later, so you sent him to school. You are surprised when he tells the doctor about his testicular pain and become extremely anxious at the thought of an operation. You worry about the effect this will have on his pubertal development and future fertility. You are reluctant to agree to any surgery without discussing with your husband, and you want to wait until he arrives from work, which may be in a few hours' time. If a sensible explanation is given regarding the diagnosis and management, you are reassured and consent.

### Instructions for Examiner

Observation only.

## Equipment Required

None.

## Mark Scheme

| | |
|---|---|
| Introduces self to the patient and his mother | |
| Checks level of comfort/need for analgesia | |
| Asks an open question to elicit the presenting complaint | |
| Establishes details of the pain: | |
| • Site of concern, radiation—asks specifically about groin/testicular pain | |
| • Onset, timing | |
| • Associated trauma | |
| • Associated symptoms, e.g. nausea, vomiting, diarrhoea, constipation, urinary symptoms | |
| • Exacerbating and relieving factors | |
| • Is he otherwise systemically well? | |
| Past medical history | |
| Family history | |
| Drug history, including immunisations and allergies | |
| Social history, including drugs and alcohol, childcare settings, and social services input | |
| Enquires if patient or mother have any specific concerns or ideas | |
| Explains the need to examine the patient's abdomen and genitalia | |
| Explains the potential diagnosis of testicular torsion | |
| Advises urgent referral to the surgical team | |
| Ensures the patient is kept nil by mouth | |
| Explains the time-critical nature of the operation and that delay can result in permanent complications | |
| Offers an information leaflet | |
| Reassures the patient that outcomes are usually good with timely surgery | |
| Sensitively discusses and manages the patient's expectations and concerns | |
| Summarises the discussion and answers any further questions | |

Total    /**23**

## Learning Points

Always remember to ask about testicular symptoms when a patient presents with abdominal pain. Failure to consider testicular torsion can result in delayed detorsion, with significant complications, e.g. reduced fertility and testicular loss. Rates of salvage of the testis decrease from 90% at six hours to <10% at 24 hours.

## References

https://cks.nice.org.uk/scrotal-pain-and-swelling

Sharp VJ, Kieran K, Arlen AM. Testicular torsion: diagnosis, evaluation, and management. *American Family Physician* 2013;**88**:835–40.

# Chapter 3 **Examinations**

# The Examination Station

An examination station is a real gift of a station and an opportunity to collect a lot of easy marks. It is sensible to think of the station in three parts: the opening, the examination itself, and the closing of the station. There will be marks for ensuring the comfort and dignity of the patient. We have used the mnemonic WIPER to remind you of these:

- Wash your hands.
- Introduce yourself to the patient.
- Permission to examine.
- Expose the patient appropriately.
- Reposition.

Remember to thank the patient and help with dressing and repositioning if required. You may be required to present your findings or management plan at this stage. The examination itself should be slick and well rehearsed. It should be complete and each aspect recognisable to the examiner. Practise rehearsing your examination both silently and by voicing your findings as you go.

You are very unlikely to be asked to simply perform an examination. You may be asked to teach an examination, or you may have to perform an examination and then provide a diagnosis and appropriate management to the patient. The patient/student is likely to be primed with specific questions regarding this.

## 3.1 **Hand Trauma**

### Instructions for Candidate

A 45-year-old builder has cut his hand on a glass window during a house renovation. Please perform a focused assessment, examine the wound, and discuss the management with him.

### Mark Scheme Breakdown

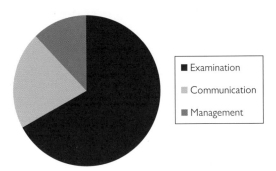

■ Examination
■ Communication
■ Management

**Figure 3.1.1** Hand trauma mark scheme breakdown.

### Instructions for Actor

You are a 45-year-old builder. You have cut your right hand on a metal girder which you were cutting whilst you were removing it from a house four hours ago. You washed the wound under a tap. The wound is on your right index finger on the palmar side. You cannot bend the tip of your finger.

You are uncertain of your tetanus status but think you had a full course many years ago. You are fit and well, with no allergies. You are in a lot of pain and would like some analgesia; you were given paracetamol in triage. You think the wound contains metal shards. You are right-handed and a keen bass guitarist.

### Equipment Required

Local anaesthetic, needle, and syringes.
X-ray of hand (Fig. 3.1.2).
Dressing and sling.

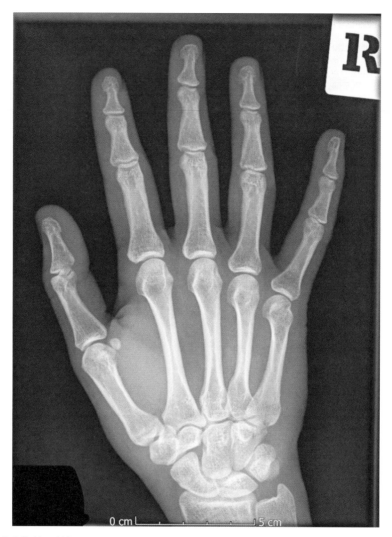

**Figure 3.1.2** Hand X-ray.

## Mark Scheme

| | |
|---|---|
| Washes hands, introduces self to the patient, seeks permission to examine, exposes and repositions the patient to sit opposite | |
| Offers analgesia | |
| Confirms key elements of the history: | |
| • When and how, laceration or crush | |

| | |
|---|---|
| • Right- or left-handed, occupation, and hobbies | |
| • Previous injury and function | |
| • Tetanus status, allergies | |
| Inspection: | |
| • Swelling, lacerations, deformity, foreign bodies | |
| Gross function: | |
| • Asks the patient to make a fist and extend the fingers | |
| Palpation: | |
| • Palpates all bones, muscles, and tendons (notes tenderness on palpation and sensation of glass in wound) | |
| Vascularity: | |
| • Assesses general colour, capillary refill time (CRT) nail bed, and radial and ulnar pulses (performs Allen's test if concerned about perfusion) | |
| Sensory function: | |
| • Radial nerve (first web space) | |
| • Median nerve (index finger) | |
| • Ulnar nerve (little finger) | |
| • Digital nerves (either side of finger laterally) | |
| Motor function: | |
| • Radial nerve: wrist extension against resistance | |
| • Median nerve: opposition of thumb and little finger | |
| • Ulnar nerve: adduction, hold paper between fingers and try to remove | |
| Tendons (general): | |
| • Notes any pain on resisted flexion (e.g. due to lacerations and flexor tendon sheath infections) | |
| Thumb: | |
| • Flexor pollicis longus (FPL): isolates the tip of the thumb and asks the patient to flex passively and actively against resistance | |
| Finger flexors: | |
| • Flexor digitorum profundus (FDP): isolates and flexes the distal tip of the finger passively and actively against resistance | |
| • Notes weakness of the index finger | |

| | |
|---|---|
| • Flexor digitorum superficialis (FDS): immobilises other fingers, so they cannot use common muscle in forearm and can only use FDS, and flexes passively and actively against resistance | |
| Finger extensors: | |
| • Asks the patient to extend all fingers (lift off flat surface individually) | |
| • Checks central slip (*Elson's test*): places the patient's hand flat on the table, with fingers over the table's edge, with the metacarpophalangeal joint (MCPJ) flexed. Extends each finger individually against resistance at proximal interphalangeal joint (PIPJ) | |
| Wrist: | |
| • Flexors: flexes the wrist and feels tendons, passively and actively against resistance | |
| • Extensors: extends the wrist passively and actively against resistance | |
| States would explore the wound under local anaesthetic | |
| Explains the likely diagnosis of FDP laceration and need for surgery | |
| Suggests appropriate management: | |
| • X-ray hand to look for metal foreign body | |
| • Confirm tetanus status with GP, may need booster | |
| • Referral to plastics for exploration, wound washout and repair | |
| Ensures the patient's comfort and dignity | |
| Thanks the patient and asks if further questions | |

Total    **/33**

## Learning Points

This is a common OSCE station. It will involve an examination, as well as knowledge of anatomy, management, and communication elements. Be well versed in the Department of Health tetanus guideline, wound care advice, local anaesthetic doses, and when antibiotics are required.

You may be asked questions by the examiner or a student regarding anatomy such as the central extensor slip or FDS/FDP. Fig. 3.1.3 shows the anatomy of the extensor tendons of the finger, including the central (middle) slip.

This may be a teaching station and you could have to teach the examination and answer questions. It may have more of a management focus and involve explaining the injury and management to the patient or making a referral to a colleague.

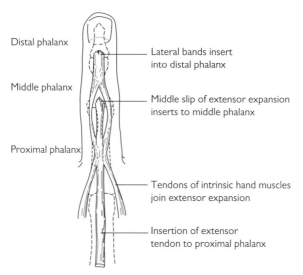

Distal phalanx

Lateral bands insert
into distal phalanx

Middle phalanx

Middle slip of extensor expansion
inserts to middle phalanx

Proximal phalanx

Tendons of intrinsic hand muscles
join extensor expansion

Insertion of extensor
tendon to proximal phalanx

**Figure 3.1.3** Central (middle) slip.

Reproduced with permission from Fig 9.10 Wounds, fractures and orthopaedics in Oxford handbook Emergency Medicine by Jonathan P. Wyatt, Robin N. Illingworth, Colin A. Graham, Kerstin Hogg, Colin Robertson, and Michael Clancy. Oxford University Press. ISBN 9780199589562.

*Tetanus Guidance*

Public Health England offers guidance about immunisation recommendations for clean and tetanus-prone wounds in Chapter 30 of the *Green Book* (see references below). The treatment that is recommended depends on the wound type and the patient's previous immunisation status.

# References

https://assets.publishing.service.gov.uk/government/uploads/system/uploads/attachment_data/file/846040/Greenbook_chapter_30_Tetanus.pdf

https://assets.publishing.service.gov.uk/government/uploads/system/uploads/attachment_data/file/849464/Tetanus_tetanus__prone_injury_poster.pdf

https://assets.publishing.service.gov.uk/government/uploads/system/uploads/attachment_data/file/849460/Tetanus_quick_guide_poster.pdf

## 3.2 **Cardiovascular**

### Instructions for Candidate

Perform a cardiovascular examination on this patient who has been having palpitations and breathlessness that started two hours ago. Present your findings to the patient and briefly advise them of treatment options.

### Mark Scheme Breakdown

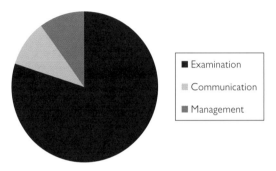

**Figure 3.2.1** Cardiovascular mark scheme breakdown.

### Instructions for Actor

You are a 43-year-old man and became aware of your heart racing two hours ago. You have no chest pain and are normally fit and well. You had six pints of lager on a work night out yesterday. You have not eaten anything today and feel light-headed when standing. You feel a little breathless on exertion. Once the treatment options are explained, ask whether this will happen again and if there is anything that can prevent it.

### Instructions for Examiner

Once the candidate has completed the examination, present them with the ECG.

### Equipment Required

ECG (Fig. 3.2.2).

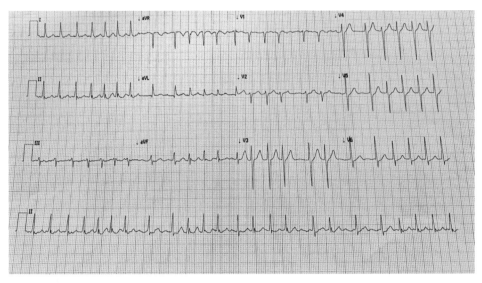

**Figure 3.2.2** ECG case 3.2.

## Mark Scheme

| | |
|---|---|
| Washes hands, introduces self, seeks permission to examine, exposes and repositions patient to 45° | |
| End of the bed inspection: | |
| • Inspects the room for clues: presence of glyceryl trinitrate (GTN) spray, $O_2$, drugs | |
| • Notes if the patient looks well, comfortable at rest, scars, permanent pacemaker (PPM), and ticking | |
| Hands: | |
| • Looks at, and feels the hands for temperature, colour, cyanosis, nicotine staining, Janeway lesions, and Osler's nodes | |
| • Looks at the nails for splinter haemorrhages, Quincke's sign, and clubbing | |
| Arm: | |
| • Takes the radial or brachial pulse; notes the rate, rhythm, and volume | |
| • Asks for BP | |
| Face: | |
| • Inspects for pallor, malar flush, mitral facies, syndromic facies, and dentition | |
| • Inspects the eyes for pallor, corneal arcus, and xanthelasma | |

| | |
|---|---|
| • Inspects the tongue and lips for central and peripheral cyanosis | |
| Neck: | |
| • Assesses the carotid pulse. Comments on character, i.e. slow-rising (aortic stenosis) or collapsing (aortic regurgitation) | |
| • Checks the jugular venous pressure (JVP) | |
| Chest inspection: | |
| • Inspects the axilla | |
| • Looks for chest deformity, asymmetry, scars, PPM, and gynaecomastia | |
| Chest palpation: | |
| • Apex | |
| • Feels for heaves and thrills | |
| • Checks for signs of a PPM | |
| Chest auscultation: feels the carotid pulse throughout | |
| • Listens in the four areas for murmurs and added sounds in inspiration and expiration | |
| • Rolls the patient onto his left lateral, using the bell to listen to mitral valve in expiration and for radiation into axilla | |
| • Sits the patient forward to 45° and listens to aortic valve at left sternal edge in expiration | |
| • Listens for crackles at lung bases | |
| Completes the examination: | |
| • Feels for sacral oedema and ankle oedema | |
| • Palpates the abdomen for abdominal aortic aneurysm (AAA), checks peripheral pulses | |
| Thanks the patient and offers help to get dressed | |
| Correctly interprets the ECG as atrial fibrillation (AF) and comments on the rate | |
| Explains the diagnosis of AF to the patient | |
| Briefly outlines treatment options of either direct current cardioversion (DCCV) or chemical cardioversion | |
| Allows time for questions from the patient and answers appropriately | |
| Confirms the management plan and closes the consultation | |

Total    /**30**

## 3.3 **Knee**

### Instructions for Candidate

Please examine this 72-year-old gentleman who has presented with a hot, painful, swollen knee and inform the patient of the likely diagnosis and the next stage of his management.

### Mark Scheme Breakdown

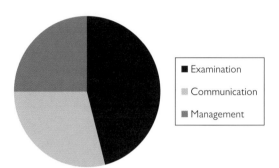

**Figure 3.3.1** Knee mark scheme breakdown.

### Instructions for Actor

You are a 72-year-old man whose left knee became swollen, red, hot, and painful yesterday. This morning, you were barely able to move your leg and you feel generally unwell. Your range of movement is extremely limited, and you will scream out if the candidate is not considerate in their examination. You have type 2 diabetes mellitus and hypertension, for which you take medications. You walk 1–2 miles per day and are not keen on hospitals. When the doctor explains the diagnosis, you are worried but happy to stay for treatment. If the candidate does not explain the diagnosis well and the importance of staying for a washout, you will try to leave and ask for oral antibiotics.

### Instructions for Examiner

Observation only.

### Equipment Required

None.

## Mark Scheme

| | |
|---|---|
| Washes hands, introduces self to the patient, seeks permission to examine, exposes and repositions the patient | |
| Offers analgesia | |
| Look (initially with the patient standing, looking bilaterally, front, and back): | |
| • Looks for scars, swelling, valgus/varus deformity, and colour change (knee looks red and swollen) | |
| • Notes the gait (unable to fully weight-bear) | |
| Feel: | |
| • Temperature (notes warmth) | |
| • Tenderness: feels with the knee in 90° flexion. Palpates around the patella, tibia, femoral condyles, head of the fibula, and joint line | |
| • Effusion: performs the tap test and/or stroke test (notes a large effusion) | |
| • Palpates the popliteal fossa for swelling, e.g. Baker's cyst/aneurysm | |
| Move: | |
| • Active: straight leg raise, flexion, and extension (notes limited range of movement due to pain) | |
| • Passive: flexion, extension, and hyperextension; simultaneously feels for crepitus | |
| States special tests are not indicated | |
| Asks for a full set of observations | |
| Examines both sides (accept if states would examine good side first) | |
| States would examine the joint above and below | |
| Thanks the patient and offers help to get dressed, ensures comfort and dignity | |
| Explains the likely differentials: septic arthritis, gout, bursitis | |
| Explains the plan to the patient: | |
| • Bloods tests (FBC, CRP, blood cultures) and aspiration of knee | |
| • Knee X-ray | |
| • IV antibiotics | |
| • Orthopaedic referral | |

| | |
|---|---|
| Allows time for questions and answers appropriately | |
| Recognises the patient's reluctance. Explains the importance of treatment and complications of untreated septic arthritis | |
| Negotiates with the patient to stay for treatment | |
| Maintains good rapport and communication | |

Total    **/24**

## 3.4 **Shoulder**

### Instructions for Candidate

Please take a focused history, examine this patient's shoulder, and explain to them the diagnosis and management.

### Mark Scheme Breakdown

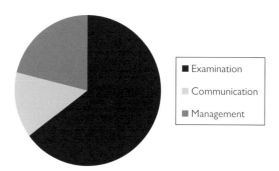

**Figure 3.4.1** Shoulder mark scheme breakdown.

### Instructions for Actor

You are a 44-year-old right-handed rugby player. Whilst playing today, you have taken a tackle and fallen to the ground, landing on your left shoulder. You now have pain and reduced range of movement in your left shoulder. You are anxious to know when you can return to sport.

On examination, you are tender over your left acromioclavicular joint (ACJ) and have noticed a lump at the end of your clavicle. It is painful to move the shoulder in any direction but feels particularly unstable when you move your arm across your body, and this makes the end of your collar bone more prominent. You have no numbness and have full strength in your hand/elbow. You have no previous shoulder injuries and are normally fit and well.

### Instructions for Examiner

Reinforce findings: visible lump distal clavicle, horizontal instability, disruption increased on adduction. Provide X-ray of shoulder (Fig. 3.4.2).

### Equipment Required

X-ray of shoulder (Fig. 3.4.2).

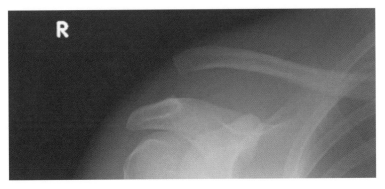

**Figure 3.4.2** X-ray of shoulder case 3.4.

Reproduced with permission from Fig 12.36.12 from Fractures and dislocations of the shoulder girdle, Oxford Textbook of Trauma and Orthopaedics (2nd Edition) by Christopher Bulstrode, James Wilson-MacDonald, Deborah M. Eastwood, John McMaster, Jeremy Fairbank, Parminder J. Singh, Sandeep Bawa, Panagoitis D. Gikas, Tim Bunker, Grey Giddins, Mark Blyth, David Stanley, Paul H. Cooke, Richard Carrington, Peter Calder, Paul Wordsworth, and Tim Briggs. Oxford University Press. ISBN 9780199550647.

## Mark Scheme

| | |
|---|---|
| Washes hands, introduces self to the patient, seeks permission to examine, exposes and repositions the patient to stand | |
| Offers analgesia | |
| Look (from all angles, including axilla): | |
| • Inspects for wasting of pectorals and deltoids | |
| • Inspects for scars, swelling, bony contours, arm position, and prominent ACJ | |
| • Inspects for winged scapula: (weak serratus anterior, supplied by long thoracic nerve) | |
| Feel: | |
| • Temperature | |
| • Palpates from sternoclavicular joint, ACJ, anterior joint line, posteriorly over acromion, scapula, and down proximal humerus | |
| • Notes prominent distal clavicle and tenderness over ACJ | |
| Move: | |
| • Assesses actively and then passively whilst feeling for crepitus | |
| • Flexion, extension, abduction (supraspinatus), adduction | |
| • Internal rotation (subscapularis), external rotation (tests against resistance to assess infraspinatus and teres minor) | |
| • Notes all movements are uncomfortable and that the clavicle is displaced superiorly and posteriorly on adduction | |

| | |
|---|---|
| Special tests: | |
| • Gerber's lift-off test | |
| • Emptying can test | |
| • Drop test | |
| • Neer's test for impingement | |
| • Apprehension test | |
| Assesses sensation: axillary nerve over sergeant's stripe, plus sensation in radial, ulnar and median nerve distribution | |
| Assesses the motor component of radial, ulnar, and median nerves | |
| Assesses pulses | |
| Thanks the patient and offers help to get dressed, ensures comfort and dignity | |
| Correctly interprets the X-ray: ACJ disruption | |
| Explains the diagnosis of ACJ disruption to the patient appropriately | |
| Explains the management: | |
| • Broad arm sling and analgesia | |
| • Follow-up review with physiotherapy and fracture clinic | |
| • Most are managed conservatively, but possibility of requiring surgery | |
| • Advises no sport until reviewed, likely three weeks at least | |
| Answers the patient's questions and summarises consultation | |

Total    /**28**

## 3.5  **Hip**

### Instructions for Candidate

Please take a focused history surrounding today's events, examine the patient's hip, and explain to the patient the likely diagnosis and management.

### Mark Scheme Breakdown

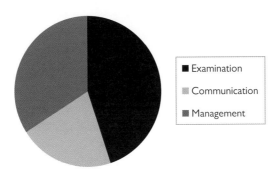

**Figure 3.5.1**  Hip mark scheme breakdown.

### Instructions for Actor

You are a 15-year-old keen footballer. Whilst playing football today, you shot a goal and felt an intense pain in your left hip. This was followed by a severe shooting pain. You are now unable to weight-bear and have restricted movements in that hip. You have no previous injuries. If asked, you have had a general mild ache in the left hip following exercise for several months.

### Instructions for Examiner

Provide pelvic X-ray (Fig. 3.5.2).

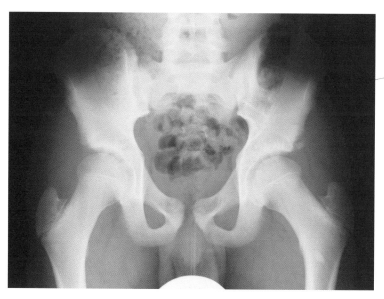

**Figure 3.5.2** Pelvic X-ray.

Reproduced with permission from Fig 85.1 from case 85 Musculoskeletal Imaging cases by Mark W. Anderson and Stacy E. Smith. Oxford University Press. ISBN 9780195394375.

## Equipment Required

Pelvic X-ray (Fig. 3.5.2).

## Mark Scheme

| | |
|---|---|
| Washes hands, introduces self to the patient, seeks permission to examine, exposes and repositions the patient | |
| Offers analgesia | |
| Look (patient standing): | |
| • Inspects for scars, wasting, curved spine, and leg position and length | |
| • Assesses the gait | |
| • Performs the Trendelenburg test to assess abductors | |
| Feel (patient lying down): | |
| • Palpates for tenderness over the greater trochanter and femoral head, and palpates prominces of pelvis, eliciting tender over the AIIS | |
| Measures leg length | |

| | |
|---|---|
| Move: | |
| • Assesses flexion and extension (whilst standing) | |
| • Assesses abduction and adduction | |
| • Assesses internal and external rotation | |
| Performs Thomas fixed flexion deformity test | |
| Checks pulses and sensation | |
| States would like to examine the joints above and below the knee | |
| Thanks the patient and offers help to get dressed | |
| Explains the likely diagnosis: avulsion fracture of AIIS | |
| Provides appropriate explanation about what this is and why it happens | |
| Outlines the immediate plan: X-ray to confirm diagnosis | |
| Advises on further management: | |
| • Rest and crutches | |
| • Analgesia | |
| • No sport for six months or until advised by orthopaedics | |
| • Physiotherapy | |
| • Paediatric fracture clinic follow-up | |
| • Occasionally need surgery | |
| Answers questions and summarises | |

Total    **/25**

# Learning Points

*Muscle Insertion Sites in Decreasing Order of Frequency of Avulsion Fracture*

- **Ischial tuberosity**: hamstrings.
- **Anterior inferior iliac spine**: rectus femoris.
- **Anterior superior iliac spine**: sartorius.
- **Superior corner of pubic symphysis**: rectus abdominis.
- **Lesser trochanter**: iliopsoas.

These injuries commonly occur in football, gymnastics, and athletics due to sprinting, jumping, kicking, or twisting. Avulsion fractures occur commonly in adolescents as the physis is the weakest portion of the immature skeleton. They occur between puberty and 25 years. The mean age of occurrence is 13.8 years.

*Presentation*

- Popping or snapping sensation.
- Low-grade pain, often for several months, preceding injury due to apophysitis.
- Point tenderness over the site.
- Possibly swelling.

*Management*

- Conservative vs surgical. Surgery leads to similar outcomes but is sometimes required in athletes or if displacement of fracture fragments is >2 cm.
- Radiographs are the mainstay of diagnosis.
- Occasionally ultrasound scan (USS), CT, or MRI are needed if the injury has not been detected or for surgical planning.
- Generally, management involves a brief period of rest, followed by protected weight-bearing, physiotherapy with progressive stretching and strengthening, and then a gradual return to sports.

# References

http://www.ncbi.nlm.nih.gov/pmc/articles/PMC2465275/table/tbl1/
https://pedemmorsels.com/pelvic-avulsion-fractures
https://www.youtube.com/watch?v=hy--bGxreAY

## 3.6 **Abdominal**

### Instructions for Candidate

You have seen a 22-year-old male with a history of 24 hours of central abdominal pain which has now become severe sharp right iliac fossa (RIF) pain, worse on movement. He feels sick and has not eaten for two days. He has low-grade fever and is mildly tachycardic at 90 bpm. He has no past medical or surgical history, is on no medications, and has no allergies. The patient has had bloods sent, but no results are available yet. He has a negative urine dip.

Please examine the patient, and explain the likely diagnosis and management. Please then refer the patient to the appropriate specialty using the phone provided.

### Mark Scheme Breakdown

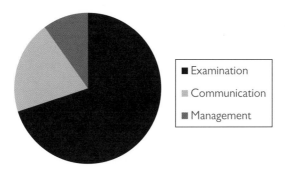

- Examination
- Communication
- Management

**Figure 3.6.1** Abdominal mark scheme breakdown.

### Instructions for Actor

*The Patient*

You are generally tender all over, but when examined in the lower right abdomen, it is very tender and you flinch. It hurts even more when the candidate lets go. You feel hot, sweaty, and nauseated.

When the candidate explains the likely diagnosis is appendicitis, you ask for pain relief (if not already offered) and understand the need for surgical review. You have no further questions.

*Surgical registrar (SpR)*

You are the SpR on call. You answer the phone to take the referral. You are a bit grumpy as you have patients to review on the ward and want to be in theatre. You decline to see the patient until the blood results are back. If the candidate communicates well that the patient is peritonitic and blood results do not alter the diagnosis or management, you will reluctantly accept the patient. If they do not communicate well, you will not come and see the patient until the blood results are back.

## Instructions for Examiner

At two minutes before the end, prompt the candidate to make a referral.

## Equipment Required

Telephone.

## Mark Scheme

| | |
|---|---|
| Washes hands, introduces self to the patient, seeks permission to examine, exposes and repositions the patient to lie flat | |
| Offers analgesia | |
| End of bed inspection: | |
| • Does the patient look well/in pain/SOB/jaundiced? Are there obvious scars or distended veins? | |
| • Medical paraphernalia: diet, drips, medications, stoma bags, catheter, drains | |
| Hands: | |
| • Assesses temperature and colour | |
| • Inspects the nails for clubbing, leuconychia, or koilonychia and checks capillary refill | |
| • Inspects the hands for Dupuytren's contractures, palmar erythema, and liver flap | |
| Arm: | |
| • Checks radial and brachial pulses and notes the rate, rhythm, and volume. Notes if a fistula is present | |
| Face: | |
| • Inspects the eyes for pallor, jaundice of sclera, corneal arcus, and xanthelasma | |
| • Looks for central cyanosis and peripheral cyanosis | |
| • Inspects the mouth for ulcers, candida, angular stomatitis, and glossitis | |
| Neck: | |
| • Assesses the JVP; checks for lymphadenopathy, particularly Virchow's node in left supraclavicular fossa | |
| Chest: | |
| • Inspects for gynaecomastia, spider naevi, and body hair distribution | |
| *Abdominal examination* | |

| | |
|---|---|
| Inspection: | |
| • Looks for scars, stoma, masses (look from side), striae, peristalsis (in obstruction), distension, bruising, and caput medusa | |
| Palpation (observes the patient's face for signs of discomfort): | |
| • Initially light palpation in nine zones and then deeper to feel for masses | |
| • Assesses for rigidity, guarding, and rebound tenderness | |
| • Palpates the liver and spleen and ballots the kidneys | |
| • Checks for the presence of AAA | |
| • Notes RIF tenderness with guarding, rigidity, and rebound tenderness | |
| Percussion: | |
| • Percusses over the liver and spleen and for signs of shifting dullness | |
| Auscultation: | |
| • Listen for bowel sounds and renal bruits | |
| Inspects the ankles for oedema | |
| States would examine the hernial orifices and external genitalia, and perform a per rectum (PR) exam | |
| Thanks the patient and offers help to get dressed | |
| States would like to review the observation chart and perform a urine dipstick | |
| Ensures patient comfort and dignity | |
| Explains the likely diagnosis is appendicitis and will need surgery | |
| Will ask the surgeons to review and take over patient's care | |
| Answers the patient's questions and demonstrates good rapport | |
| Calls the surgical registrar and makes a good referral | |
| Negotiates effectively to ensure the patient is reviewed promptly, even without blood results | |
| Demonstrates good communication and remains calm and polite | |

Total    /**31**

# Learning Points

The nuance of this station is to test your negotiation skills, alongside your examination technique, in order to optimise the care of your patient in a timely manner. Atema et al. (2015) concluded that 'no WBC count or CRP level can safely and sufficiently confirm or exclude the suspected diagnosis of acute appendicitis in patients who present with abdominal pain of five days or less in duration'. The diagnosis is a clinical one and warrants surgical review. Occasionally, imaging will then be required.

## Reference

Atema JJ, Gans SL, Beenen LF, *et al*. Accuracy of white blood cell count and C-reactive protein levels related to duration of symptoms in patients suspected of acute appendicitis. *Academic Emergency Medicine* 2015;**22**:1015–24.

## 3.7 **Cranial Nerves**

### Instructions for Candidate

Mrs Howard has a sudden-onset severe headache which came on whilst having a cigarette in a break from hoovering at work an hour ago. She has never had such a severe headache before, despite suffering from migraines many years ago. She has tried simple analgesia, but it has not improved. She is bothered by the light, has double vision, and is keen to lie down in the dark. She suffers from hypertension and type 2 diabetes.

Please examine Mrs Howard, and provide a differential diagnosis and management plan.

### Mark Scheme Breakdown

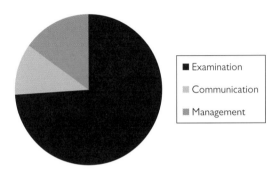

**Figure 3.7.1** Cranial nerves mark scheme breakdown.

### Instructions for Actor

You have the worst headache ever and just want to lie down in the dark and not open your eyes. You have previously had migraines, but this is completely different—you have not had a headache this severe and have no aura or associated migraine symptoms. You are struggling to keep your left eyelid open and you have double vision. You feel sick and your neck is stiff. You had a bad headache last week, but it settled after some painkillers and a sleep. You take amlodipine and metformin and smoke 20 cigarettes per day. You would really like some pain relief.

### Instructions for Examiner

If the candidate states they will test hearing, gag reflex, corneal reflex, and colour vision inform them they are normal and move on.

If the candidate does not provide a diagnosis and management plan, prompt them to do so one minute before the end of the station. Ask them to confirm their differential diagnosis.

# Equipment Required

Ophthalmoscope.
Cotton wool.
Tendon hammer.
Tuning fork.
Tongue depressor.

# Mark Scheme

| | |
|---|---|
| Washes hands, introduces self to the patient, seeks permission to examine, exposes and repositions the patient to sit opposite | |
| Offers analgesia | |
| Olfactory nerve: | |
| • Asks about changes in sense of taste or smell | |
| Optic nerve: | |
| • Asks about changes in vision | |
| • Checks visual acuity (VA) with a Snellen chart | |
| • Mentions assessing colour vision with Ishihara plates | |
| • Performs fundoscopy | |
| • Assesses visual fields | |
| • Assesses pupillary response to light and accommodation and checks for relative afferent pupillary defect (RAPD) | |
| Oculomotor, trochlear, and abducens nerves: | |
| • Uses 'H' pattern to look for conjugate eye movements, nystagmus, and diplopia | |
| Trigeminal nerve: | |
| • Assesses sensation in the three division areas and compares both sides | |
| • Assesses the muscles of mastication | |
| • Assesses corneal reflex (afferent) and jaw jerk reflex | |
| Facial nerve: | |
| • Inspects for facial asymmetry | |
| • Assesses the muscles of facial expression | |

| | |
|---|---|
| Vestibulocochlear nerve: | |
| • Assesses gross hearing function | |
| • If hearing loss is detected, performs Rinne's and Weber's tests (512 Hz fork) | |
| Glossopharyngeal and vagus nerves: | |
| • Assesses for speech quality and volume | |
| • Assesses the palate for elevation and the uvula for deviation | |
| • Offers to test the gag reflex | |
| Accessory nerve: | |
| • Assesses sternocleidomastoid and trapezius muscles | |
| Hypoglossal nerve: | |
| • Assesses the tongue for fasciculation, wasting, and deviation | |
| Thanks the patient and ensures comfort and dignity | |
| Correctly identifies signs: left ptosis and third nerve palsy with diplopia | |
| Explains possible diagnosis to patient and advises urgent CT head with angiogram and neurosurgical review | |
| Gives appropriate differential to examiner: posterior communicating artery aneurysm | |
| Explains appropriately to the patient and answers questions | |

Total    /**27**

# Learning Points

The cranial nerve (CN) examination is worth practising. A well-prepared candidate will make it easy for the examiner to give marks. Some techniques are outlined in this section.

### Oculomotor (CN III), Trochlear (CN IV), and Abducens (CN VI) Nerves

Ask if the patient can see your one upheld finger. Keeping the patient's head still, ask them to follow your finger with their eyes, moving in an 'H' pattern. Look for conjugate eye movements, nystagmus, and diplopia.

Remember (LR6SO4)3—the lateral rectus is innervated by CN VI, and the superior oblique by CN IV, and CN III innervates the other muscles of the eye.

### Trigeminal Nerve (CN V)

The sensory branches ($V_1$, $V_2$, and $V_3$) supply the face, which is divided into three areas (forehead, cheek, and lower jaw). Ask the patient to close their eyes, and with a cotton wool tip, touch on the three division areas and compare bilaterally to assess sensation.

The motor branches supply the muscles of mastication. Ask the patient to clench their teeth. Palpate the temporalis and masseter muscles. Ask the patient to open their mouth and resist you closing it to test the pterygoids.

Branches of the trigeminal nerve are also responsible for the corneal reflex (afferent) and jaw jerk reflex.

### Facial Nerve (CN VII)

CN VII supplies the muscles of facial expression. Ask the patient to raise their eyebrows, screw up their eyes, blow their cheeks out, and grin. It also supplies the stapedius, which dampens hearing, and so injury to this branch results in hyperacusis.

The facial nerve also supplies taste sensation to the anterior two-thirds of the tongue.

### Vestibulocochlear Nerve (CN VIII)

For gross assessment of hearing, cover one of the patient's ears, rub your fingers together by one ear, whisper a number in the other ear, and ask them to repeat it. If there is a hearing deficit, Rinne's and Weber's tests can be performed to determine if it is a sensorineural or a conduction problem. Use the 512 Hz tuning fork.

- **Rinne's test**: place the vibrating tuning fork next to the ear, then on the mastoid process. Which is loudest? Normally, air conduction is greater than bone conduction. If bone conduction is greater than air conduction, this suggests conductive loss.
- **Weber's test**: place the fork in the middle of the patient's forehead and ask if it sounds louder in one ear. In conductive loss, it is heard loudest in the affected ear. In sensorineural loss, it is heard loudest in the unaffected ear.

### Glossopharyngeal (CN IX) and Vagus (CN X) Nerves

These are usually tested together. CN IX supplies the sensation of taste to the posterior third of the tongue. It also forms the afferent limb of the gag response.

CN X forms the efferent limb of the gag response. A lesion causes asymmetrical palate elevation and uvula deviation (pulled to the normal side). It can also result in dysarthria and difficulty in making high-pitched noises due to vocal cord paralysis.

### Accessory Nerve (CN XI)

CN XI supplies the sternocleidomastoids and trapezius. Test by asking the patient to shrug and turn their head laterally against resistance.

### Hypoglossal Nerve (CN XII)

CN XII supplies most of the muscles of the tongue. Inspect the tongue for fasciculation and wasting. Ask the patient to protrude the tongue, then inspect for deviation. If there is a lesion in CN XII, the tongue will deviate towards the affected side.

## 3.8 **Lower Limb Neurology**

### Instructions for Candidate

Mr Drummond presents with lower back pain and leg weakness. He is a 45-year-old lorry driver who previously had a prolapsed lumbar disc and sciatica. He lifted some heavy boxes last week and has had worsening pain and weakness since.

Please examine the patient and provide a differential diagnosis and management plan to the patient.

### Mark Scheme Breakdown

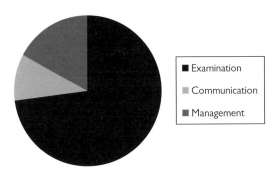

**Figure 3.8.1** Lower limb neurology mark scheme breakdown.

### Instructions for Actor

You find it incredibly hard to get from standing to lying and to lift your legs onto the bed. You have a slight foot drop when you walk, which you had not noticed, but when mentioned, you recall that you did trip over yesterday.

On examination, you have weakness of ankle dorsiflexion and inversion, as well as weakness of hallux extension and knee flexion. You have sensory loss to your posterior thigh, lower leg, and foot, sparing the medial side of your lower leg. You have absent ankle jerk, but your knee jerk is present. Your pain is much worse on straight leg raise and causes pain to shoot down the back of your leg.

You are too embarrassed to mention, but yesterday you had an episode of urinary incontinence and you have been unable to get an erection for two days. If examined, you have reduced perineal sensation.

When the candidate explains the diagnosis, you are very concerned regarding permanent erectile dysfunction and weakness. You are concerned you will not be able to drive and earn an income.

### Instructions for Examiner

If the candidate asks to assess the perineum, tell the candidate the patient has normal anal tone, but reduced sensation.

If the candidate does not provide a diagnosis and management plan, prompt them to do so one minute before the end of the station.

## Equipment Required

Neuro tips.
Tuning forks.
Tendon hammer.

## Mark Scheme

| | |
|---|---|
| Washes hands, introduces self to the patient, seeks permission to examine, exposes and repositions the patient | |
| Offers analgesia | |
| Inspection: | |
| • With the patient standing, inspects anteriorly and posteriorly for wasting, fasciculation, asymmetry, scars, positioning, and contractures | |
| • Assesses gait and heel–toe walking | |
| • Romberg's test for proprioception | |
| Tone: | |
| • Assesses tone and clonus (<2 beats normal) | |
| Power: | |
| • Assesses power at the hip (flexion, extension, abduction, adduction) | |
| • Assesses power at the knee (flexion, extension) | |
| • Assesses power at the ankle (dorsiflexion, plantarflexion, inversion, eversion) | |
| • Assesses power of the big toe (extension) | |
| Coordination: | |
| • Performs the heel–shin test | |
| Reflexes: | |
| • Tests the patellar reflex | |
| • Tests the ankle jerk reflex | |
| • Tests the plantar response | |

| | |
|---|---|
| Sensation: | |
| • Tests each modality according to dermatomes, and compares both sides with the patient's eyes closed | |
| • Assesses light touch | |
| • Assesses painful sensations | |
| • Assesses temperature | |
| • Assesses vibration with a 128 Hz tuning fork | |
| • Assesses proprioception at the big toe | |
| Ensures comfort and dignity | |
| Thanks the patient and offers help to get dressed | |
| Correctly identifies clinical signs: | |
| • Motor loss: weak ankle dorsiflexion, ankle inversion, hallux extension, and knee flexion | |
| • Sensory loss: posterior thigh, lower leg, and foot, sparing the medial side of lower leg | |
| • Reflexes: absent ankle jerk | |
| Asks about incontinence, erectile dysfunction, and loss of perineal sensation | |
| States would assess perineal sensation and anal tone | |
| Explains the diagnosis of possible cauda equina syndrome L4/5 radiculopathy with disc disease | |
| States the need for urgent MRI spine and review by the spinal/neurosurgical team | |
| Answers the patient clearly and empathetically | |

Total      /**30**

# Learning Points

This section includes summary points for the components of the lower limb neurology examination.

*Power*

Table 3.8.1 summarises the movements of the lower limb, along with the associated muscle groups and innervation, that are used in the assessment of power.

**Table 3.8.1** Summary of assessment of power of the lower limb

| Movement | Muscle | Nerve | Nerve root |
|---|---|---|---|
| Hip flexion | Iliopsoas | Femoral nerve | L1/2 |
| Hip extension | Gluteus maximus | Inferior gluteal nerve | L5/S1 |
| Hip abduction | Gluteus medius and minimus | Superior gluteal nerve | L4/5/S1 |
| Hip adduction | Adductors | Obturator nerve | L2/3/4 |
| Knee flexion | Hamstrings | Sciatic nerve | L5/S1 |
| Knee extension | Quadriceps | Femoral nerve | L3/4 |
| Ankle dorsiflexion | Tibialis anterior | Deep peroneal nerve | L4/5 |
| Ankle plantarflexion | Gastrocnemius | Posterior tibial nerve | S1/2 |
| Ankle inversion | Tibialis posterior | Tibial nerve | L4/5 |
| Ankle eversion | Peroneus longus and brevis | Superior peroneal nerve | L5/S1 |
| Big toe extension | Extensor hallucis longus | Deep peroneal nerve | L5 |

*Medical Research Council (MRC) Power Grading*

- **0**: no movement.
- **1**: flicker of movement.
- **2**: movement with gravity eliminated.
- **3**: movement against gravity.
- **4**: movement against resistance, but incomplete.
- **5**: normal power for age and sex.

*Reflexes*

- **Knee**: L3/4, femoral nerve.
- **Ankle**: S1/2, tibial nerve.
- **Plantar response or Babinski reflex**: upper motor neurone lesions cause upgoing plantars.

*Reflex Grading*

- **0**: absent.
- **+/–**: present with reinforcement.
- **+**: just present.
- **++**: brisk normal.
- **+++**: exaggerated response.

*Sensation*

Test each modality according to dermatomes, and compare both sides, with the patient's eyes closed, demonstrating on their sternum first.

*Dermatomes*

Figs. 3.8.2 and 3.8.3 demonstrate the dermatomes from the anterior and posterior aspects, respectively.

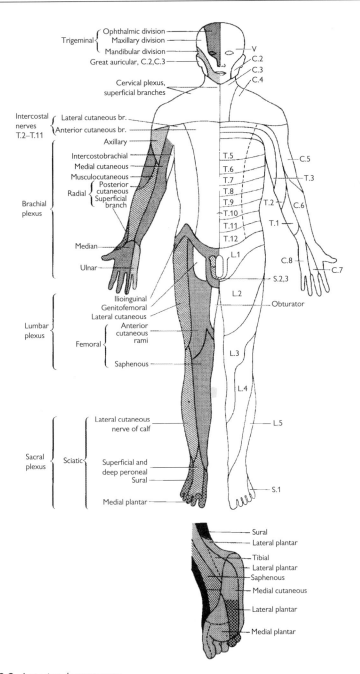

**Figure 3.8.2** Anterior dermatomes

From Fig 8.23 from Major Trauma in Oxford Handbook of Emergency Medicine by Jonathan P. Wyatt, Robert G. Taylor, Kerstin de Wit, and Emily J. Hotton. Oxford university press. ISBN 9780198784197.

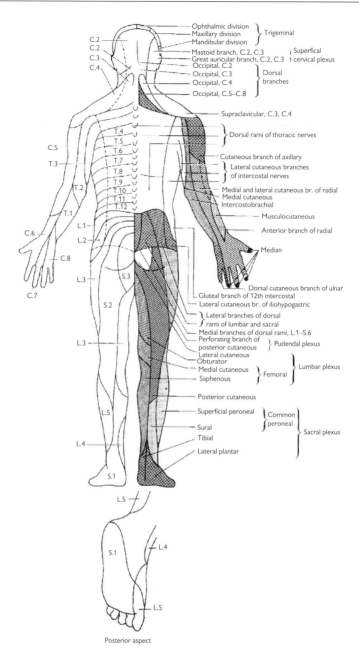

**Figure 3.8.3** Posterior dermatomes

From Fig 8.23 from Major Trauma in Oxford Handbook of Emergency Medicine by Jonathan P. Wyatt, Robert G. Taylor, Kerstin de Wit, and Emily J. Hotton. Oxford university press. ISBN 9780198784197.

*Upper Limb Neurology*

This station could easily be adapted to assess upper limb neurology. Included in this section are brief summaries of different components of the upper limb neurology examination. Figs. 3.8.2 and 3.8.3 demonstrate the anterior and posterior aspects, respectively, of the dermatomes of the upper limb.

*Power*

(See Table 3.8.2.)

**Table 3.8.2** Summary of assessment of power of the upper limb

| Movement | Muscle | Nerve | Nerve root |
|---|---|---|---|
| Shoulder abduction | Deltoid | Axillary nerve | C5 |
| Shoulder adduction | Latissimus dorsi | Thoracodorsal nerve | C6/7/8 |
| Shoulder adduction | Pectoralis major | Medial and lateral pectoral nerves | C5–T1 |
| Elbow flexion | Biceps | Musculocutaneous nerve | C5/6 |
| Elbow extension | Triceps | Radial nerve | C7 |
| Wrist flexion | Flexor carpi ulnaris | Ulnar nerve | C8 |
| Wrist flexion | Flexor carpi radialis | Median nerve | C7 |
| Wrist extension | Extensor carpi radialis | Radial nerve | C6/7 |
| Finger flexion | FDS and FDP | Median nerve, ulnar nerve | C8 |
| Finger extension | Extensor digitorum | Posterior interosseous nerve from radial | C7 |
| Finger abduction | Dorsal interossei | Ulnar nerve | T1 |
| Thumb abduction | Abductor pollicis brevis | Median nerve | T1 |

*Pronator Test*

Ask the patient to put their arms out in front, with their palms up and eyes shut. In cerebellar disorders, the arm rises; in weakness, it will pronate and drift. You may see pseudoathetosis (fingers wriggle/drift due to a proprioception disorder).

*Reflexes*

- **Biceps**: C5/6.
- **Triceps**: C7.
- **Supinator**: C6.
- **Fingers**: C8.

## 3.9 **Cerebellar**

### Instructions for Candidate

This 56-year-old lady has attended with dizziness, difficulty walking, and slurred speech. Her BP is 180/90 mmHg. Please perform a focused cerebellar examination and provide feedback on your differential and management plan to the patient.

### Mark Scheme Breakdown

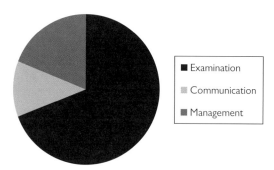

**Figure 3.9.1** Cerebellar mark scheme breakdown.

### Instructions for Actor

You are a 56-year-old lady with a history of hypertension and hypercholesterolaemia. You have had two hours of double vision; you feel off balance and are struggling to walk, and your speech is slurred and odd. You have no history of inner ear disorders and have no tinnitus or headache.

### Instructions for Examiner

Give the following examination findings to candidate: dysarthria with slurred, staccato speech, diplopia, vertical nystagmus, and wide-based ataxic gait.

### Equipment Required

Tendon hammer.

# Mark Scheme

| | |
|---|---|
| Washes hands, introduces self to the patient, seeks permission to examine, exposes and repositions the patient | |
| Offers analgesia | |
| Upper limb: | |
| • Upper limb tone, power and reflexes | |
| • Dysdiadochokinesia | |
| • Finger–nose test: past pointing and intention tremor | |
| • Cerebellar drift (arms out, palms facing up; will pronate and drift up in cerebellar dysfunction) | |
| • Dysmetria: arms out in front, tap palm, and arms will spring up | |
| Face: | |
| • Inspects for nystagmus and head titubation | |
| Speech: | |
| Assesses for dysarthria: 'British constitution', 'Baby hippopotamus', staccato and slurred speech | |
| Lower limbs: | |
| • Assesses lower limb tone, power and reflexes | |
| • Assesses heel–shin coordination | |
| Thanks the patient and offers help to get dressed | |
| **Explains the differential diagnosis and management plan to the patient** | |

NB Up to 2 marks are available for actions in bold.

Total /**16**

# Learning Points

Table 3.9.1 can help you to differentiate peripheral from central vertigo.

**Table 3.9.1** Peripheral and central vertigo

| Peripheral vertigo | Central vertigo |
| --- | --- |
| • Benign paroxysmal positional vertigo (BPPV)<br>• Vestibular neuritis<br>• Acute labyrinthitis<br>• Otitis media<br>• Cholesteatoma | • Transient ischaemic attack (TIA)/stroke<br>• Acoustic neuroma<br>• Cerebellopontine tumour |
| Sudden | Gradual: space-occupying lesion (SOL). Very sudden: stroke/TIA |
| Severe nausea and vomiting | Mild nausea and vomiting |
| Auditory symptoms: fullness, tinnitus, hearing loss | Usually no auditory symptoms (except acoustic neuroma) |
| Exacerbated by head movement | Head movement has little effect |
| No neurology, except horizontal nystagmus—remains same direction, fatigues with fixation | Neurology: dysarthria, diplopia, dysdiadochokinesia, dysmetria, hemiparesis, vertical nystagmus (bidirectional, does not fatigue, persists with fixation), ataxia |
| Head impulse test positive—i.e. catch-up saccade after bringing head briskly back to centre from 20° | No saccade |
| | Abnormal test of skew |

Adapted from Table 7.3 Differences between peripheral and central vertigo and Table 7.4 Differences between peripheral and central nystagmus, and Table 7.5 Peripheral and central causes of vertigo in *Revision notes for MCEM part B* by Victoria Stacey. Oxford University Press. ISBN 978-0-19-959277-7.

# Reference

https://cks.nice.org.uk/vertigo#!topicSummary

## 3.10 **Ankle and Foot**

### Instructions for Candidate

Mr Curtis is a 45-year-old builder. He was walking his dog when he felt a sudden snap and pain in his left ankle. He now is unable to fully weight-bear and his ankle is swollen. Please examine him and explain to the patient the diagnosis and management.

### Mark Scheme Breakdown

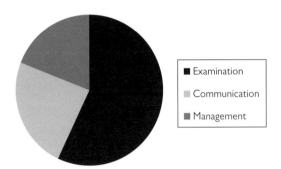

**Figure 3.10.1** Ankle and foot mark scheme breakdown.

### Instructions for Actor

You are very physically active. You were walking your dog yesterday on a five-mile trail when you felt a sudden snap and severe pain in your left ankle. You are very worried about having time off work. You now have a very swollen and painful ankle and are struggling to walk on it. You want it dealt with as soon as possible as you cannot afford not to work. You take prednisolone 5 mg once daily (OD) for polymyalgia rheumatica (PMR) but are otherwise healthy.

### Instructions for Examiner

Observation only.

### Equipment Required

None.

# Mark Scheme

| | |
|---|---|
| Washes hands, introduces self to the patient, seeks permission to examine, exposes and repositions the patient to 45° after assessing the gait | |
| Offers analgesia | |
| Look: | |
| • Inspects the gait | |
| • Looks for asymmetry, deformities, scars, swelling, and bruising | |
| Feel: | |
| • Temperature | |
| • Tenderness—palpates over bones, joints, ligaments, and tendons and demonstrates good knowledge of surface anatomy of the foot and ankle | |
| • Notes a palpable step and tenderness over the Achilles tendon | |
| • Palpates pulses | |
| Move: | |
| • Assesses active and passive movements | |
| • Ankle dorsiflexion, plantarflexion, inversion, and eversion | |
| • Toe flexion and extension | |
| Assesses movements of foot joints | |
| Performs Simmonds–Thompson calf squeeze test | |
| States intention to examine both ankles and the knee | |
| Thanks the patient and offers help to get dressed | |
| Explains the diagnosis of ruptured Achilles tendon | |
| Explains the management plan: | |
| • Treat with equinus cast initially | |
| • USS to confirm the diagnosis and site of rupture | |
| • Referral for orthopaedic review in clinic | |
| • Discharge with analgesia, VTE prophylaxis, and crutches | |
| Answers any questions and summarises the consultation | |

Total    /**21**

# Learning Points

*The Simmonds–Thompson Calf Squeeze Test*

Lie the patient prone, with the feet and ankle off the end of the bed. Squeeze the calf. Failure to plantarflex the foot indicates Achilles tendon rupture. Beware a partial rupture which may elicit plantarflexion. If in doubt, organise an USS.

## 3.11  Eye

### Instructions for Candidate

A 58-year-old lady has been brought in with a headache, vomiting, and a red, painful eye. Please examine her and outline the next steps in her management and make the appropriate referral.

### Mark Scheme Breakdown

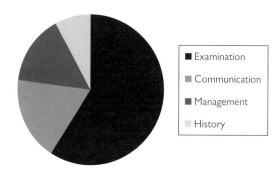

- Examination
- Communication
- Management
- History

**Figure 3.11.1** Eye mark scheme breakdown.

### Instructions for Actor

*Patient*

You are a 58-year-old librarian and developed a painful eye this evening when reading in a dimly lit room. You also have blurred vision and a headache. You normally wear glasses as you are long-sighted. You have vomited twice at home and once in the ED. You have mild asthma, for which you take Atrovent® and salbutamol, and take oxybutynin for bladder control.

*Ophthalmology Senior House Officer (SHO)*

You have 30 minutes left on your shift and still have two patients to review. You have never had to deal with an acute closed-angle glaucoma before and you are uncertain whether this is the correct diagnosis. You think it sounds more like a migraine and are not convinced by the stated examination findings. You are very reluctant to accept the patient and suggest that they are brought back to clinic in the morning. If the candidate states that they will escalate to your senior, you will concede to review them tonight.

### Equipment Required

Snellen chart.
Ophthalmoscope.
Image of eye (Fig. 3.11.2).

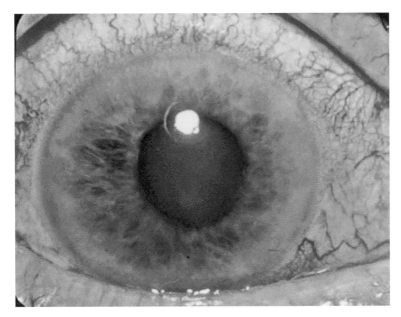

**Figure 3.11.2** Image of eye in case 3.11.

Reproduced from Fig 5.26 from Oxford Handbook of Clinical Specialties (10 edn) by Andrew Baldwin, Nina Hjelde, Charlotte Goumalatsou, and Gil Myers. Oxford University Press. ISBN 9780198719021.

## Mark Scheme

| | |
|---|---|
| Washes hands, introduces self to the patient, seeks permission to examine, exposes and repositions the patient for optimal assessment | |
| Offers analgesia and anti-emetic | |
| Elicits the history and establishes that the symptoms worsened on entering a darkened room | |
| Establishes the patient is hypermetropic | |
| Elicits drug history and establishes that the patient takes two anticholinergic drugs | |
| VA: | |
| • Assesses VA of both eyes with glasses and pinhole and the Snellen chart at 6 m | |
| • Assesses near vision: ability to read paper, etc. | |
| Inspection: | |
| • External: looks for ptosis, asymmetry, proptosis, positioning, squint, and photophobia | |
| • Lids: looks for swelling, ectropion, and blepharitis | |
| • Notes asymmetry and lacrimation | |
| • Gross inspection: comments on hazy cornea and circumcorneal erythema | |

| | |
|---|---|
| Pupils: | |
| • Records pupil size, shape, and direct and consensual responses to light and accommodation | |
| • Comments on fixed, semi-dilated, ovoid pupil | |
| • Notes RAPD | |
| Eye movements: | |
| • Checks eye movements using 'H' pattern | |
| • Observes for diplopia, nystagmus, and ptosis | |
| Assesses visual fields | |
| Fundoscopy: | |
| • Correctly sets up ophthalmoscope | |
| • Checks the red reflex | |
| • Examines the four quadrants of the retina, disc, macula, and fovea | |
| Palpates the globe and states would measure the intraocular pressure | |
| States would use the slit-lamp to examine the eye | |
| Assesses colour vision | |
| Explains the diagnosis of acute angle-closure glaucoma to the patient | |
| Explains to the patient the next steps in management: | |
| • 500 mg acetazolamide IV | |
| • 0.5% timolol drops topically | |
| • 2% pilocarpine drops—every 15 minutes (both eyes) | |
| • Urgent referral to ophthalmology for laser peripheral iridotomy | |
| Refers to ophthalmology and outlines the key features | |
| Does not concede for next-day review | |
| Remains professional, but firm. Suggests escalation to SHO's senior if no agreement to review the patient this evening | |
| Ensures the patient's comfort and dignity throughout | |
| Thanks the patient and closes station appropriately | |

Total    /**34**

## 3.12 **Maxillofacial**

### Instructions for Candidate

Friends have brought in a 19-year-old man after an altercation on a night out. He was allegedly punched and kicked in the head and face. Please assess his injuries and outline a management plan.

### Mark Scheme Breakdown

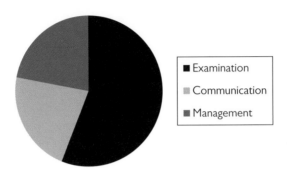

**Figure 3.12.1** Maxillofacial mark scheme breakdown.

### Instructions for Actor

You are a 19-year-old student. You were out drinking with friends when you were involved in a fight over a spilled drink. You have had six pints of beer and several shots and are heavily intoxicated. Three men attacked you and you were punched several times in the face and kicked in the jaw. You are struggling to open your mouth and have an abnormal bite when asked.

### Equipment Required

X-ray mandible (Fig. 3.12.2).

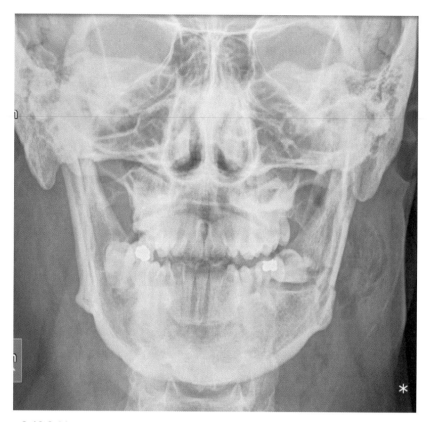

**Figure 3.12.2** X-ray mandible.

## Mark Scheme

| | |
|---|---|
| Washes hands, introduces self to the patient, seeks permission to examine, exposes and repositions the patient for optimal assessment | |
| Offers analgesia | |
| Ensures the airway is safe before proceeding further | |
| Briefly clarifies the mechanism of injury | |
| Checks NICE head injury red flags | |
| States would first complete an ABCDE assessment and ensure no C-spine injury | |
| Inspects and palpates the scalp: | |
| • Looks for lacerations, haematomas, and foreign bodies | |

| | |
|---|---|
| Palpates the supraorbital and infraorbital rims: | |
| • Assesses for tenderness, steps, crepitus, and surgical emphysema | |
| • Checks sensation above and below the rims and on the cheek | |
| Palpates over the zygoma, nose, maxilla, and mandible. Checks sensation on the chin | |
| Palpates the temporomandibular joint (TMJ) on mouth opening (if possible) | |
| Inspects for Battle's sign behind the ears | |
| Mouth: | |
| • Inspects dentition, looks for internal trauma or lacerations to gums | |
| • Pulls forwards on teeth to check for shift of the maxilla | |
| • Confirms abnormal bite. If possible, puts fingers inside the patient's cheek and asks them to clench their teeth | |
| Nose: | |
| • Inspects for septal deviation or haematoma | |
| Eyes: | |
| • Inspects and palpates the globe | |
| • Everts the eyelids to check for trauma and foreign bodies | |
| • Checks eye movements, asks about diplopia | |
| • Checks VA | |
| Ears: | |
| • Uses an otoscope to look for perforation of tympanic membrane or trauma | |
| Outlines the next steps in the management—orthopantomogram (OPG)/facial X-ray (accept CT head as alternative) | |
| Correctly interprets the X-ray as a fracture to left ramus of the mandible | |
| Management plan: | |
| • Referral to maxillofacial surgeons | |
| • Keeps the patient nil by mouth and offers analgesia | |
| • Discusses management of the assault—asks whether it has been reported to the police | |
| Thanks the patient and closes the station appropriately | |

Total    /**27**

# Chapter 4 **Teaching**

# The Teaching Station

Teaching forms a large part of the OSCE. Expect at least two teaching stations and note that other stations, such as the resuscitation or practical skills stations, may have small teaching components, e.g. talking through chest drain insertion in a trauma scenario, teaching how to suture whilst performing it yourself, or teaching a patient how to use an inhaler.

The exam is fair and assesses routine things we should be competent to perform daily. Make a list of all the practical procedures you have to perform and write down a stepwise approach of how you would teach them.

In Section 4.1, you will find a generic mark scheme which you can apply to any teaching station. It is important not to miss the marks that are common to any teaching station at the beginning and end of the scenario. You can still pass a station or at least achieve a higher score with buffering of the cumulative overall mark if the main element does not go well, as long as you tick the generic marks. Section 4.2 outlines some additional points that are relevant to a teaching station that involves patient contact. The rest of the chapter provides specific scenarios to work through, along with a complete mark scheme.

At the end of this chapter, you will find a list of some other possible teaching stations you should prepare (see Section 4.15).

## 4.1 **Generic Mark Scheme**

A significant portion of the mark scheme is allocated to generic actions that can be applied to most teaching stations.

## Mark Scheme

| | |
|---|---|
| Introduces self | |
| Clarifies what the student already knows | |
| Asks the student what they want to learn | |
| Agrees the learning objectives to be covered in this teaching session | |
| Demonstrates the skill/examination | |
| Asks student to perform the skill | |
| Reinforces correct technique and highlights relevant learning points | |
| Plans future sessions and encourages ongoing practice | |
| Signposts to further reading materials or resources | |
| Gives the student the opportunity to ask questions | |
| Summarises and ends the session | |

## Learning Points

In addition to the generic mark scheme outlined, there may be marks for consenting the patient, confirming the correct site, or discussing the requirement for the procedure. If the instruction is to teach a procedure, there will be a point for post-procedure care (see Chapter 5). There may also be a point for demonstrating good communication with the student or patient. Examples of this will be given in the sections that follow within this chapter.

## 4.2 **Examination Mark Scheme**

When teaching an examination, there are certain components relating to the patient that you should add into the generic teaching mark scheme that was described in Section 4.1. These additional components are outlined in the following mark scheme.

### Mark Scheme

| | |
|---|---|
| Introduces self and the student to the patient | |
| Asks the patient's permission to be examined and be the subject of the teaching session | |
| Reassures the patient that the examination findings and management plan will be explained at the end of the session | |
| Demonstrates the examination or skill | |
| Asks the student to perform the examination | |
| Reinforces learning and corrects the student's technique in real time | |
| Thanks the patient and offers help to get dressed | |

### Learning Points

Always remember to be respectful and mindful of the patient in the scenario, as you would in real life.

In the OSCE, it is likely that you will not have time to do a full four-stage teaching technique that is common to certain life support courses. Consider which components of the procedure you will focus on, then demonstrate and explain the steps as you go along, and then allow the student to have a go, talking it through in real time.

## 4.3 **Respiratory Examination**

### Instructions for Candidate

A third-year medical student has taken a history from a 45-year-old man with a productive cough and fever, but otherwise normal vital signs. The patient has had a rapid swab test with a negative result for Covid-19. The student has asked for your help to examine the patient and to plan ongoing care.

### Mark Scheme Breakdown

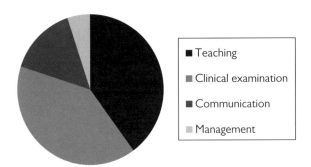

**Figure 4.3.1** Respiratory examination mark scheme breakdown.

### Instructions for Actor

*Third-Year Medical Student*

You are a third-year medical student; you have learnt the theory of clinical examinations but have not yet examined a patient. You will ask the doctor to teach you how to perform a respiratory examination. You will ask them to perform the examination and explain what they are doing and will then have a go yourself.

You have some questions regarding the management of this patient: how can you grade the severity of the chest infection? Can the patient be discharged?

*Patient*

You have a productive cough, feel mildly breathless on exertion, and have a fever. You are not confused. You want to know if you need a CXR and whether you need antibiotics. You consent to be the subject of a teaching session with the medical student.

### Instructions for Examiner

When the patient has been examined, please confirm that the patient has coarse crackles in their left base.

## Equipment Required

None.

## Mark Scheme

| | |
|---|---|
| Introduces self to student | |
| Clarifies who they are, what their previous experience of the examination has been, and what they would like to learn and achieve today | |
| Agrees on the objectives for the session | |
| Introduces self and student to the patient | |
| Asks the patient's permission to be examined and be the subject of the teaching session | |
| Reassures the patient that the examination findings and management plan will be explained at the end of the session | |
| Washes hands, introduces self, seeks permission to examine the chest, exposes and repositions the patient to 45° | |
| Demonstrates the examination: | |
| Inspection: | |
| • Assesses the patient's general well-being, notes any scars and the use of accessory muscles | |
| • Looks for the presence of drugs or inhalers, $O_2$ therapy, sputum pots, and cigarettes | |
| Hands: | |
| • Looks and feels hands for temperature, colour, and nicotine staining. Examines the nails for clubbing | |
| • Checks for carbon dioxide ($CO_2$) retention flap and tremor (e.g. due to salbutamol) | |
| Arm: | |
| • Assesses radial and brachial pulses, and notes the rate, rhythm, and volume | |
| • Measures the RR | |
| Face: | |
| • Looks at the eyes for pallor. Looks under the tongue for central cyanosis and lips for peripheral cyanosis | |
| Neck: | |
| • Assesses the JVP, any lymphadenopathy, and tracheal position | |

| | |
|---|---|
| Anterior chest: | |
| • Inspects for chest deformity (e.g. barrel chest, pectus excavatum), asymmetry, scars, and use of accessory muscles | |
| • Palpates the chest, assesses chest expansion, and locates the apex beat | |
| • Demonstrates tactile fremitus and vocal resonance | |
| • Percusses the chest in all areas | |
| • Auscultates the chest in all areas | |
| Completes the examination by checking the patient's peak flow or reviewing the peak flow diary | |
| Asks the student to perform the examination of the posterior chest | |
| Reinforces learning and corrects the student's technique in real time | |
| Thanks the patient and offers help to get dressed | |
| Discusses the findings with the student (coarse crackles at the left base) and the diagnosis of left lower lobe (LLL) pneumonia | |
| Explains to the patient they have a left-sided pneumonia | |
| Answers the patient's questions regarding CXR and antibiotics | |
| Asks the student if there are any questions | |
| Explains the CURB65 score to assess severity of pneumonia | |
| Explains that the patient has normal observations and appears well. His CURB65 score is likely 0, so the patient can be discharged with oral antibiotics | |
| Summarises the session | |
| Suggests further resources to access, e.g. books and online video tutorials | |
| Sets a time for a further session and suggests new learning objectives | |

Total    /**33**

# Learning Points

You should be guided by the student about which components you teach. For example, they may wish to focus on examining the chest and cover the peripheral examination another time. Or you could demonstrate the peripheral examination and how to examine the posterior chest and then ask them to examine the anterior chest.

This station may have an actor with reportable signs and may have a management component to it. The student is likely to have primed questions for you regarding the examination and management of the patient. Make sure you know relevant clinical scoring tools, such as the CURB65, as this is an obvious question for the student to ask you. Be aware, though, that the CURB65 tool is not validated in people with COVID-19.

## References

https://www.nice.org.uk/guidance/ng165
https://www.nice.org.uk/guidance/NG173

## 4.4 **Cranial Nerve Examination**

### Instructions for Candidate

A Foundation Year 1 (F1) doctor has seen a patient with a facial droop and is uncertain of the diagnosis. She has asked for your help to teach her a CN examination, confirm the clinical signs, and help her manage the patient.

### Mark Scheme Breakdown

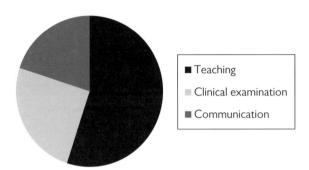

**Figure 4.4.1** Cranial nerve examination mark scheme breakdown.

### Instructions for Actor

*F1 Doctor*

You are an F1 doctor. You are not confident in CN examinations but have examined a patient with a facial droop. You ask the doctor to teach you how to perform an examination of CN II to VII. Ask them to explain what they are doing and what their findings are. You have some questions regarding the management of this patient: how can you differentiate a Bell's palsy from a stroke? What is the management of this patient?

*Patient*

You have a right-sided facial droop. You understand the diagnosis and management when it is explained to you.

### Equipment Required

None.

# Mark Scheme

| | |
|---|---|
| Introduces self to student | |
| Clarifies who they are, what their previous experience of the examination has been, and what they would like to learn and achieve today | |
| Agrees on the objectives for the session | |
| Introduces self and student to the patient | |
| Asks the patient's permission to be examined and be the subject of the teaching session | |
| Reassures the patient that the examination findings and management plan will be explained at the end of the session | |
| **CN II:** | |
| • Asks about changes in vision | |
| • Tests visual acuity with a Snellen chart | |
| • Performs fundoscopy | |
| • Tests visual fields with a red pin | |
| • Checks direct and consensual pupillary reflexes and accommodation, and assesses for RAPD | |
| • Checks colour vision with Ishihara plates | |
| **CN III, IV, VI:** | |
| • Assesses eye movements | |
| • Asks the patient if they have double vision and where | |
| • Notes if there is an extraocular muscle palsy or nystagmus | |
| **CN V:** | |
| • Assesses the sensory branches. Asks the patient to close their eyes, then uses cotton wool to test the three division areas. Compares both sides of the face. Repeats the assessment using a sharp tip | |
| • Assesses the motor branches to the muscles of mastication. Asks the patient to clench their teeth. Palpates temporalis and masseter. Asks the patient to open their mouth against resistance to test the pterygoids | |
| • Assesses the corneal reflex and jaw reflex | |
| **CN VII:** | |
| • Inspects the muscles of facial expression for asymmetry | |
| • Asks the patient to copy facial movements (raise eyebrows, screw eyes closed, blow out the cheeks, toothy smile) | |

| | |
|---|---|
| • States that CN VII is also responsible for the sensation of taste to the anterior two-thirds of tongue | |
| • States that CN VII supplies the stapedius which is responsible for dampening of hearing, and lesions can result in hyperacusis | |
| Asks the student to perform the examination | |
| Reinforces learning and corrects the student's technique in real time | |
| Discusses the findings with the student: the patient is unable to corrugate forehead. The patient has a lower motor neurone (LMN) facial nerve palsy | |
| Explains that in an upper motor neurone (UMN) palsy, the forehead is spared as the frontalis has bilateral innervation from corticospinal fibres | |
| Thanks the patient | |
| Explains to the patient they have a Bell's palsy and what this means | |
| Asks the student if there are any questions | |
| Answers the student's questions: | |
| • Advises 50 mg prednisolone OD for ten days | |
| • Discusses eye care: artificial tears, protective glasses, patch at night | |
| Explains the prognosis: related to initial severity. Approximately 85% show recovery by three weeks | |
| Summarises the session | |
| Suggests further resources to access, e.g. books and online video tutorials | |
| Sets a time for a further session and suggests new learning objectives | |

Total    /**35**

## Learning Points

NICE does not recommend antiviral treatments alone for Bells palsy alone but concedes that there may be a small benefit when combined with steroids, and suggests that specialist advice is sought. An example dose would be prednisolone 60 mg OD plus valaciclovir 1000 mg three times daily (TDS).

NICE suggests two possible steroid regimes:

• Prednisolone 50 mg daily for ten days, or
• Prednisolone 60 mg daily for five days, followed by a daily reduction in dose of 10 mg.

## Reference

https://cks.nice.org.uk/bells-palsy#!background

## 4.5 **Paediatric Elbow X-Ray Interpretation**

### Instructions for Candidate

Please teach this Foundation Year 2 (F2) doctor how to interpret a paediatric elbow X-ray.

### Mark Scheme Breakdown

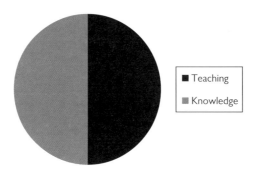

**Figure 4.5.1** Paediatric elbow X-ray interpretation mark scheme breakdown.

### Instructions for Actor

You are an F2 doctor who has just rotated to the ED. You have never been taught how to interpret paediatric elbow X-rays before. You have just seen a nine-year-old boy after a fall from a skateboard and you want to check his X-ray is normal prior to discharge. The child has had analgesia.

### Instructions for Examiner

Observation only.

# Equipment Required

Normal elbow X-ray (lateral and anteroposterior views) of nine-year-old child (Figs. 4.5.2 and 4.5.3).

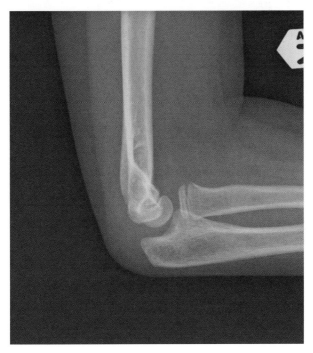

**Figure 4.5.2** Elbow X-ray lateral.

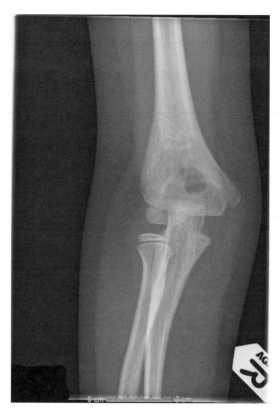

**Figure 4.5.3** Elbow X-ray AP.

## Mark Scheme

| | |
|---|---|
| Introduces self to junior doctor | |
| Establishes the F2's previous experience and knowledge | |
| Asks if there are any specific learning needs | |
| Agrees on the objectives for the session | |
| Asks for a brief history and mechanism of injury | |
| Checks the patient requires no immediate treatment (analgesia) and is neurovascularly intact | |
| Checks the patient's details and time on the X-rays are correct | |
| Describes the terms and explains the need to check: | |
| • Fat pads | |
| • Radiocapitellar line | |

| | |
|---|---|
| • Anterior humeral line | |
| • Ossification centres | |
| Explains the significance of CRITOL | |
| Asks the F2 doctor to interpret the X-ray | |
| Reinforces key learning points | |
| Correctly interprets the elbow X-ray as normal | |
| Checks if the F2 has any questions or concerns | |
| Answers questions appropriately | |
| Agrees a plan for ongoing learning | |
| Suggests further resources to access, e.g. books and online tutorials | |
| Good rapport and teaching style | |

Total    **/20**

## Learning Points

There are six ossification centres in the elbow, which appear in a reproducible order, although there may be variability in the age at which they appear. The order can be remembered using the mnemonic CRITOL. The ages are approximate, but easy to recall (Table 4.5.1).

**Table 4.5.1** Ossification centres of the elbow

| Ossification centre | Approximate age (years) at appearance |
|---|:---:|
| Capitellum | 1 |
| Radial head | 3 |
| Internal (medial) epicondyle | 5 |
| Trochlea | 7 |
| Olecranon | 9 |
| Lateral epicondyle | 11 |

Knowledge of CRITOL is important to prevent missing an injury. Essentially, if the trochlea is present, then you should be able to see the medial (internal) epicondyle. If it is not located medially on the X-ray, then it must be displaced. Medial epicondyle injuries require orthopaedic review and open reduction and internal fixation (ORIF). The typical mechanism is 'a direct blow or valgus stress at the elbow and contraction of the flexor muscles'. 50% are associated with a dislocation.

# References

https://radiopaedia.org/articles/elbow-ossification?lang=gb
https://radiopaedia.org/articles/paediatric-elbow-radiograph-an-approach?lang=gb
https://dontforgetthebubbles.com/elbow-xr-interpretation/

## 4.6 **Kendrick Splint Application**

### Instructions for Candidate

You are called to the resuscitation area to help treat a 47-year-old man who has fallen from his loft. He has been assessed as part of a trauma call and is haemodynamically stable, but has an isolated femoral fracture. He has had a femoral nerve block, and your SHO wants help to apply a Kendrick splint. Please apply the splint whilst explaining the procedure to the SHO.

### Mark Scheme Breakdown

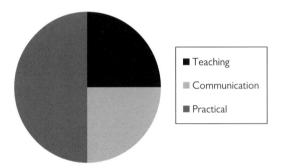

**Figure 4.6.1** Kendrick splint application mark scheme breakdown.

### Instructions for Actor

You are an SHO with some Emergency Medicine experience. You understand the principles of splint application, as you have previously used a Thomas splint, but have not used a Kendrick splint before.

### Equipment Required

Actor for splint application.
Kendrick splint.

### Mark Scheme

| | |
|---|---|
| Introduces self to SHO | |
| Clarifies what their previous experience is and discusses their learning needs | |
| Agrees on the objectives for this case | |
| Introduces self and SHO to patient, confirms patient's name, and offers analgesia | |

| | |
|---|---|
| Explains the procedure and asks permission to teach whilst performing the procedure | |
| Checks the patient's neurovascular status | |
| Ensures the femoral nerve block has been given and is working | |
| Demonstrates and explains the following steps to the SHO: | |
| • Applies the ankle hitch | |
| • Applies the thigh strap, as close to the groin as possible | |
| • Extends the traction pole and measures it against the patient's leg. Ensures the black line on the pole is level with the patient's foot. Inserts the pole into the thigh strap | |
| • Attaches the elastic knee strap | |
| • Inserts the black foot bar of the pole into the yellow loop, then pulls the red cord tight to create traction | |
| • Attaches the elastic thigh and ankle straps | |
| • Rechecks the patient's neurovascular status | |
| Covers the patient to maintain dignity and ensures he/she is comfortable | |
| Thanks the patient | |
| Provides a summary and invites questions from the SHO | |
| Arranges a further session to practise and to cover other learning needs | |
| Suggests further learning resources to access, e.g. books and online tutorials | |
| Overall communication with SHO | |

Total    /**20**

## Learning Points

There are many online demonstrations of a Kendrick splint application. Simply using the search terms 'Kendrick splint' will generate videos to watch on how to apply the splint. We found the East Midlands Emergency Medicine Educational Media (EM3FOAMed) and Prometheus videos useful. It is important to familiarise yourself with the splint, so make sure you take opportunities during work time to practise.

## References

EM3FOAMed. *How to apply a Kendrick splint*. https://www.youtube.com/watch?v=QIxzroh2rhw
Prometheusmed. *Prometheus traction splint*. https://www.youtube.com/watch?v=ZQO0Vj1rD8M

# 4.7 **Hearing Assessment**

## Instructions for Candidate

You have an F1 doctor shadowing you today. You are about to assess a patient with the presenting complaint of 'hearing loss'. Please teach the F1 how to complete an examination appropriate for this patient.

## Mark Scheme Breakdown

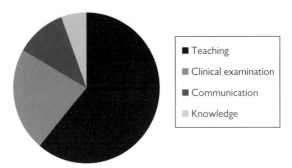

■ Teaching
■ Clinical examination
■ Communication
■ Knowledge

**Figure 4.7.1** Hearing assessment mark scheme breakdown.

## Instructions for Actor

You have hearing loss in your right ear. You are a keen sea swimmer. You have noticed some recent pain in the ear, with redness and itching around the outer ear. You often feel a pressure inside your ear like a sensation of fullness.

## Equipment Required

Otoscope.
512 Hz tuning fork.
Image showing otitis externa (Fig. 4.7.2).

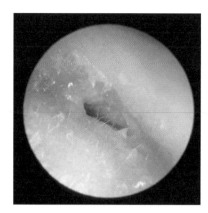

**Figure 4.7.2** Otitis externa.

Reproduced from Figure 7.23. Ear Nose & Throat. In Oxford Handbook of Clinical Specialties (10th Edn) by Andrew Baldwin, Nina Hjelde, Charlotte Coumalatsou and Gil Myers. Oxford University Press. ISBN 9780198719021.

## Mark Scheme

| | |
|---|---|
| Introduces self to the F1, checks their experience and knowledge | |
| Discusses the learning needs and agrees the objectives for today | |
| Introduces self to patient, confirms patient's name, and offers analgesia | |
| Explains the procedure and asks permission to teach whilst performing it | |
| Demonstrates and explains the components of the assessment, ensuring both sides are examined | |
| Inspection: | |
| • Looks for hearing aids, characteristic facies, scars, pre-auricular sinus, eczema, and otitis externa | |
| Palpation: | |
| • Palpates pre-, post-, and infra-auricular lymph nodes. Palpates for tenderness and swelling of the lobe, helix, tragus, and antihelix | |
| Otoscopy: | |
| • Describes the parts of the otoscope: light source, disposable attachment of correct size, handle | |
| • Explains the procedure to the patient and repositions the patient to sit comfortably | |
| • Holds the handle of the scope with the right hand to look at the right ear | |
| • Uses the other hand to pull the pinna back to straighten the canal | |
| • Looks at the external canal for wax/discharge/skin changes | |

| | |
|---|---|
| • Inspects the internal canal. Visualises the tympanic membrane and checks for the light reflex, effusion, perforation, cholesteatoma, and grommets | |
| Notes the presence of otitis externa | |
| Hearing assessment: | |
| • Assesses grossly by occluding one ear and whispering a number from 1 m away | |
| • Performs Rinne's test by placing a 512 Hz vibrating tuning fork on the patient's mastoid process. When it is no longer heard, moves it to in front of the same ear | |
| • Performs Weber's test by placing the vibrating tuning fork in the middle of the forehead. Asks the patient if it sounds equal in both ears | |
| Interprets the findings to the F1—correctly identifies conductive hearing loss in the right ear | |
| Asks the student to perform the examination. Reinforces learning and corrects the student's technique in real time | |
| Provides a summary and invites questions from the F1 | |
| Arranges further session to practise and cover other learning needs | |
| Suggests further learning resources to access, e.g. books and online tutorials | |
| Thanks the patient and explains the diagnosis | |
| Discusses the management plan with the patient | |

Total    /**24**

## Learning Points

*Rinne's Test*

Rinne's test is a screen for conductive hearing loss. In normal hearing, air conduction (AC) is greater than bone conduction (BC). If BC is greater than AC, this indicates a conductive hearing loss. In sensorineural loss, both AC and BC are equally diminished, so when Rinne's test is applied, a normal result (i.e. AC > BC) is obtained.

*Weber's Test*

Weber's test is often used alongside Rinne's test.
• In normal hearing (AC > BC): the sound of the tuning fork is the same bilaterally.
• In sensorineural hearing loss (AC > BC): the sound will be louder in the normal ear.
• In conductive hearing loss (BC > AC): the sound will be louder in the affected ear.

*Management of Otitis Externa*

• Take swabs if there is any discharge, particularly if there has been previous treatment failure.
• Prescribe suitable drops such as Gentisone®.
• After swimming or bathing, drain the ear by tilting the head laterally. Dry the external ear canal with a hairdryer; do not rub with a towel.

- Do not use ear buds to clean the ear canal. Use olive oil for wax removal.
- Review after one week if no improvement for consideration of alternative drops or aural toilet.

## References

https://gpnotebook.com/simplepage.cfm?ID=2100625427
https://cks.nice.org.uk/otitis externa#!scenarioRecommendation:6

# 4.8 Arterial Blood Gas Interpretation

## Instructions for Candidate

An F2 doctor has seen a patient in Resus and is worried by the arterial blood gas (ABG) result. Please explain the blood gas to the F2 and advise on how to manage the patient.

## Mark Scheme Breakdown

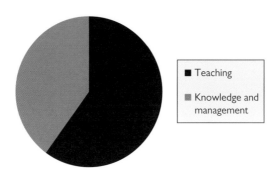

**Figure 4.8.1** Arterial blood gas interpretation mark scheme breakdown.

## Instructions for Actor

You are an F2 doctor and you have seen a patient in Resus with chronic obstructive pulmonary disease (COPD) who looks unwell. His $O_2$ saturations are 79%; he is cyanosed and tachypnoeic at 40 breaths per minute and has a GCS of 13. You have taken an ABG and given the patient a salbutamol nebuliser, but you are not sure how to interpret the ABG or how to manage the patient. You have run out of Resus in a panic to get help. A nurse remains with the patient.

If the doctor does not ask for any patient information, do not volunteer it, but steer them towards teaching you gas interpretation. If they do ask, tell them the patient's observations and that you are concerned they look awful and are peri-arrest.

## Instructions for Examiner

If the candidate expresses concern about the patient and states the need to review the patient, reassure the candidate that they may continue with the teaching session as the patient is already being reviewed by another senior doctor.

## Equipment Required

ABG results (Table 4.8.1).

**Table 4.8.1** Arterial blood gas results.

| pH | 7.21 |
|---|---|
| $pCO_2$ | 13.1 kPa |
| $pO_2$ | 7.39 kPa |
| ctHb | 137 g/l |
| $cK^+$ | 4.5 mmol/l |
| $cNa^+$ | 139 mmol/l |
| $cCa^{2+}$ | 1.18 mmol/l |
| $cCl^-$ | 96 mmol/l |
| cGlu | 9.5 mmol/l |
| cLac | 3.1 mmol/l |
| $cHCO_3^-$ | 35.2 mmol/l |
| cCr | 185 mmol/l |

## Mark Scheme

| | |
|---|---|
| Introduces self to F2, checks existing experience and knowledge | |
| Asks about the patient's clinical status, observations, and whether someone is looking after them | |
| States the need to urgently review the patient and initiate the patient's treatment first, and invites the F2 to join in | |
| Reassures the F2 that once the patient is stable, you will explain the ABG and the management | |
| Discusses the F2's learning needs and sets objectives for today | |
| Agrees to teach normal values, basic interpretation, and the acute management of the patient | |
| Teaches the normal blood pH values: 7.35–7.45 | |
| • pH <7.35 is acidaemia, pH >7.45 is alkalaemia | |
| Teaches the normal $paCO_2$ values: 4.7–6.0 kPa | |
| • Explains $CO_2 + H_2O \Leftrightarrow H^+ + HCO_3^-$ | |
| • Increased $CO_2$ pushes the equation to the right and increases $H^+$ and therefore increases acidity (decreases pH) and results in respiratory acidosis | |

| | |
|---|---|
| Teaches the normal $HCO_3^-$ values: 22–26 mmol/l | |
| • When $HCO_3$ buffers $H^+ \Rightarrow H_2O + CO_2$, therefore acid is excreted | |
| • If $H^+$ increased, $HCO_3^-$ will be used to buffer and reduce acidity. Once reserves are exhausted, $H^+$ increases and results in metabolic acidosis | |
| Teaches the normal $paO_2$ value: 11 kPa | |
| • Rough rule is $paO_2 = FiO_2 - 10$ kPa | |
| Checks understanding and provides a summary, e.g. Table 4.8.2 | |
| Asks the F2 to work through and describe the patient's gas | |
| Facilitates the student's learning and confirms it shows respiratory acidosis and why | |
| Relates the blood gas result to the clinical picture | |
| Discusses the acute management of the patient: | |
| • Recognises it is type 2 respiratory failure | |
| • Advises nebulisers, steroids, controlled $O_2$ therapy, and bilevel positive airway pressure (BIPAP) | |
| Provides a summary and invites questions from the F2 | |
| Arranges a further session to practise and address other learning needs, e.g. renal compensation and non-invasive ventilation | |
| Suggests further learning resources | |

Total /**25**

## Learning Points

Table 4.8.2 can be used as an aide memoire to help the student work out the basics of the ABG.

**Table 4.8.2** Arterial blood gas interpretation summary

| | **Acidosis** | **Alkalosis** |
|---|---|---|
| Respiratory | pH ↓<br>$CO_2$ ↑ | pH ↑<br>$CO_2$ ↓ |
| Metabolic | pH ↓<br>$HCO_3^-$ ↓ | pH ↑<br>$HCO_3^-$ ↑ |

## Reference

https://litfl.com/acid-base-disorders/

## 4.9 **Overdose Management**

### Instructions for Candidate

A Specialty Trainee Year 1 (ST1) doctor has seen a patient in Majors who is apparently drunk. However, a bottle of antifreeze has been found in his coat. The ST1 asks you for help to interpret the blood gas and to talk through how to manage the patient.

### Mark Scheme Breakdown

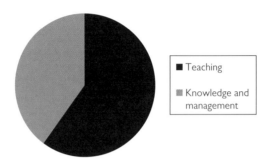

**Figure 4.9.1** Antifreeze overdose mark scheme breakdown.

### Instructions for Actor

You are an ST1 doctor and you are not familiar with managing patients with overdose. You have assessed a patient in Majors who appears to be drunk. You have taken a blood gas and have brought it to the registrar on shift to ask for advice.

You have specific questions:

- How do you interpret the blood gas?
- How do you know if the patient is just drunk or has taken antifreeze? What is antifreeze?
- How should you manage the patient? Is there an antidote? When do you give it? How does the antidote work?
- Ask how you can find information about poisons and overdoses next time you have a patient.

### Instructions for Examiner

Inform the candidate the patient is safe and being cared for and that they can continue to teach the ST1 if they ask.

### Equipment Required

ABG results (Table 4.9.1).

**Table 4.9.1** Arterial blood gas results (overdose).

| pH | 7.34 |
| --- | --- |
| $pCO_2$ | 3.02 kPa |
| $pO_2$ | 18.9 kPa |
| ctHb | 112 g/l |
| $cK^+$ | 3.3 mmol/l |
| $cNa^+$ | 138 mmol/l |
| $cCa^{2+}$ | 1.09 mmol/l |
| $cCl^-$ | 106 mmol/l |
| cGlu | 15.5 mmol/l |
| cLac | 10.0 mmol/l |
| $cHCO_3^-$ | 11.8 mmol/l |
| cCr | 56 mmol/l |

# Mark Scheme

| | |
| --- | --- |
| Introduces self, checks the ST1 doctor's existing experience and knowledge | |
| Asks about the patient's clinical status and observations, and whether someone is looking after them | |
| States the need to urgently review the patient and initiate the patient's treatment first, and invites the trainee to join in | |
| Reassures the ST1 that once the patient is stable, you will explain the ABG and the management | |
| Discusses the ST1's learning needs and sets the objectives for today | |
| Asks the ST1 to work through and describe the patient's ABG (metabolic acidosis and raised lactate) | |
| Describes the blood gas: | |
| • Metabolic acidosis with raised anion gap and raised lactate | |
| • Initially a raised osmolar gap as they absorb the alcohol, but falls later as it is metabolised | |
| • Associated hypocalcaemia and raised creatinine | |
| Teaches the ST1 how to calculate the anion gap and the osmolar gap | |

| | |
|---|---|
| Describes the typical clinical presentation of someone who has taken an antifreeze overdose | |
| Discusses the management of the patient: | |
| • A thorough ABCDE assessment, correcting problems as they are noted | |
| • Fomepizole or ethanol are the antidotes | |
| • Antidote to be given if suspect >10 g ingested, or any amount ingested and exhibiting a toxic effect | |
| Provides summary and invites questions from ST1, answers appropriately | |
| Suggests further learning resources, e.g. TOXBASE® | |
| Arranges further session to practise and address other learning needs | |

Total    /**17**

## Learning Points

*Antifreeze Overdose*

Following the ingestion of antifreeze, the patient may present inebriated, then become acidotic and tachypnoeic, and may subsequently develop coma, seizures, hypertension, and renal failure.

Antifreeze contains ethylene glycol, which is converted by alcohol dehydrogenase to glycoaldehyde and then to glycolic, glycoxylic, and oxalic acids. Glycolic acid causes marked metabolic acidosis. During this, nicotinamide adenine dinucleotide (NAD) is reduced to NADH, which decreases the conversion of lactate to pyruvate and so results in lactic acidosis.

Fomepizole inhibits alcohol dehydrogenase and reduces the conversion of ethylene glycol to glycoaldehyde. This increases the elimination half-life.

Patients may need haemodialysis in a large overdose with an ethylene glycol level >8 mmol/l, pH <7.3, and acute renal failure.

*Useful Calculations*

$$\textbf{Anion gap} = [Na^+] + [K^+] - [HCO_3^-] + [Cl^-] = 12\text{–}16$$

$$\textbf{Osmolar gap} = \text{measured osmolality} - \text{calculated osmolality}$$

$$\textbf{Calculated osmolality} = 2[Na^+] + [\text{glucose}] + [\text{urea}]$$

## References

https://lifeinthefastlane.com/tox-library/toxicant/alcohols/ethylene-glycol/
https://www.toxbase.org/poisons-index-a-z/e-products/ethylene-glycol/

## 4.10 **Suturing**

### Instructions for Candidate

You are asked by a junior doctor to help you suture a patient as they do not know how to suture a V-shaped flap. Please teach this skill and answer any questions they have. The patient sustained a clean wound from a glass window two hours ago, and their tetanus immunisation is up-to-date.

### Mark Scheme Breakdown

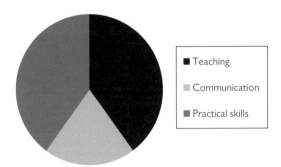

**Figure 4.10.1** Suturing mark scheme breakdown.

### Instructions for Actor

You are an SHO with some emergency medicine experience. You can do basic interrupted sutures but do not know how to approach a flap. Ask them to demonstrate how to suture the flap. When you suture the straight sides of the wound, you will need to be corrected as you do not tie the knot well.

If asked, confirm an X-ray was taken and that there is no glass *in situ*. You want to know:

• How much local anaesthetic to use.
• If tetanus immunisation is required.
• If antibiotics are required.
• More about wound care.

### Equipment Required

Actor and dummy wound.
Suturing equipment.

## Mark Scheme

| | |
|---|---|
| Introduces self to the SHO, checks their experience/learning needs, and sets objectives for session | |
| Introduces self to patient, confirms patient's name, and offers analgesia | |
| Obtains informed consent from the patient for the procedure and asks permission to teach whilst performing the procedure | |
| Confirms the X-ray has been reviewed and no glass is visible | |
| Confirms local anaesthetic has been given and is effective | |
| States the maximum dose of local anaesthetic: lidocaine 3 mg/kg | |
| Washes hands and uses sterile gloves and a drape | |
| Cleans the wound and explores depth (no structures visible, superficial wound) | |
| Selects an appropriate suture | |
| Demonstrates and explains how to suture a flap to avoid tissue necrosis at the tip | |
| Handles the instruments and tissues correctly. Uses a non-touch technique and ties a secure knot | |
| Asks the SHO to insert interrupted sutures into the side of the wound | |
| Corrects the technique and teaches the SHO how to tie a knot | |
| Disposes of sharps safely | |
| Dresses the wound | |
| Confirms tetanus status and that no booster required | |
| Answers the SHO's questions about when to give tetanus immunoglobulin or vaccine | |
| Gives wound care advice to the patient. Explains when to remove the sutures and signs of infection to look out for | |
| Answers the SHO's questions appropriately regarding antibiotics—no requirement in this case | |
| Provides summary and invites questions from the SHO | |
| Arranges further session to practise/cover other learning needs and suggests further learning resources | |
| Good patient interaction | |

Total    /22

# Learning Points

*Tetanus Guidance*

Public Health England has published guidance on immunisation for clean and tetanus-prone wounds (see Section 3.1).

*General Wound Care Guidance*

Sutures should be removed at 3–5 days on the head or face, 10–14 days over joints, and 7–10 days over other areas.

Wounds closed by glue and Steristrip® should be kept clean and dry for five days.

Once the sutures have been removed, moisturise, massage, and use sunblock to reduce scarring.

# References

https://www.nhs.uk/common-health-questions/accidents-first-aid-and-treatments/
    how-do-i-care-for-a-wound-treated-with-skin-glue/
https://www.nhs.uk/common-health-questions/accidents-first-aid-and-treatments/
    how-do-i-apply-butterfly-stitches/

## 4.11 **Intraosseous Access**

### Instructions for Candidate

Please teach this medical student how to insert an intraosseous (IO) needle.

### Mark Scheme Breakdown

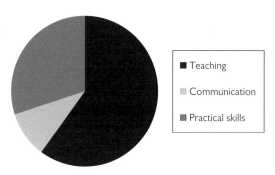

- ■ Teaching
- ▨ Communication
- ■ Practical skills

**Figure 4.11.1** Intraosseous access mark scheme breakdown.

### Instructions for Actor

You are a final-year medical student. You are keen to learn how to insert an IO needle. If not mentioned by the candidate, ask about complications, contraindications, and sites of insertion.

### Instructions for Examiner

Observation only.

### Equipment Required

EZ-IO®.
Dummy tibia.

### Mark Scheme

| | |
|---|---|
| Introduces self to the medical student | |
| Establishes previous experience and knowledge and asks if there are any specific learning needs | |
| Sets out learning objectives | |

| | |
|---|---|
| Discusses the indications and uses of IO access | |
| Discusses the contraindications | |
| Discusses the complications | |
| Discusses sites of insertion: | |
| • Proximal tibia: 2 cm below and medial to tibial tuberosity | |
| • Distal tibia: 3 cm above medial malleolus | |
| • Proximal humerus: 1 cm above greater tubercle (with arm adducted and palm resting on abdomen) | |
| • Distal femur: 3 cm above lateral condyle | |
| Discusses needle sizes | |
| Demonstrates the insertion: | |
| • Prepares equipment | |
| • Identifies landmarks | |
| • Uses local anaesthetic if the patient is concious and aware | |
| • Cleans the site of insertion | |
| • Pushes needle through skin at 90°, keeping the black line visible. Drills until feels a 'give' | |
| • Removes the needle and disposes into a sharps bin | |
| • Aspirates and then secures the IO access | |
| • Attaches a pre-flushed 3-way tap connector. Pushes fluids (± local anaesthetic) by syringe | |
| Allows medical student to practise | |
| Corrects the student's technique as appropriate | |
| Summarises the session | |
| Agrees a plan for ongoing learning | |
| Suggests appropriate learning resources | |
| Good rapport and teaching style | |

Total    **/25**

# Learning Points

*Contraindications to IO Access*

IO access is contraindicated if:

- There is infection at the insertion site.
- You cannot locate the landmarks.
- There has been previous IO access at that site within 48 hours.
- There is a fracture proximal to the insertion site.
- There is severe osteoporosis/osteogenesis.
- The patient has had orthopaedic surgery near the site.

*Complications of IO Access*

Complications include extravasation, physeal plate injury, infection/osteomyelitis, compartment syndrome, pain, dislodgement, haematoma, fracture, skin necrosis, and embolism.

## 4.12 **Bier's Block**

### Instructions for Candidate

Please teach the ST1 doctor how to perform a Bier's block. There is a 72-year-old lady with a Colles' fracture that requires manipulation. She is otherwise healthy and has been nil by mouth for six hours.

### Mark Scheme Breakdown

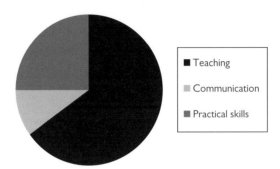

■ Teaching
▨ Communication
▩ Practical skills

**Figure 4.12.1** Bier's block mark scheme breakdown.

### Instructions for Actor

You are an ST1 doctor. You have never performed a Bier's block before. Your patient is a 72-year-old lady with a Colles' fracture which needs manipulation.

If the candidate does not mention it, ask about complications, the dose of prilocaine to use, and the recognition and management of local anaesthetic toxicity.

### Instructions for Examiner

Observation only.

### Equipment Required

Patient.
Double-cuff tourniquet.
Prilocaine.
Monitoring/resuscitation equipment.

## Mark Scheme

| | |
|---|---|
| Introduces self to junior doctor | |
| Establishes ST1's previous experience and knowledge | |
| Confirms the specific learning needs and sets the learning objectives | |
| Prepares the equipment, checks the tourniquet has no leaks | |
| Obtains informed consent from the patient and asks permission to teach whilst performing the procedure | |
| Discusses contraindications to Bier's blocks | |
| Discusses the safety requirements: two staff present, full monitoring, resuscitation equipment available, IV access in each arm | |
| Calculates the safe dose of 0.5% prilocaine: 3 mg/kg used (but max safe dose is 6 mg/kg) | |
| Talks through the steps of the procedure: | |
| • Record the patient's vital signs, noting the systolic BP | |
| • Put on the cuff and check the radial pulse is palpable | |
| • Exsanguinate the injured arm for three minutes | |
| • Inflate the double cuff to 100 mmHg over initial systolic BP, or to a maximum of 300 mmHg. Note the time the cuff was inflated | |
| • Confirm the radial pulse is now absent | |
| • Inject the prilocaine and note the time | |
| • Check the anaesthesia is effective (if inadequate after five minutes, give a 5 ml saline flush) | |
| • Remove the cannula from the injured arm and manipulate the fracture | |
| • Check the X-ray to confirm adequate manipulation | |
| • Explain the cuff must remain inflated for at least 20 minutes, for a maximum of 45 minutes | |
| • Deflate the cuff and note the time | |
| • Ensure the patient is under observation for 30 minutes before discharge | |
| • Arrange follow-up | |
| Asks the ST1 to talk through the steps and perform the procedure. Offers guidance and corrections as necessary | |

| | |
|---|---|
| Invites questions | |
| Answers the ST1's questions about toxicity appropriately | |
| Agrees a plan for ongoing learning | |
| Suggests appropriate learning resources | |
| Good teaching rapport | |

Total    **/27**

# Learning Points

*Contraindications to a Bier's Block*

Do not perform a Bier's block in patients with bilateral fractures, peripheral vascular disease, Raynaud's, a systolic BP >200 mmHg, SCD, methaemoglobinaemia, obesity, cellulitis of the limb, lymphoedema, an open fracture, or crush injury. It is also not indicated in patients who are confused or uncooperative.

The RCEM has published guidance on the use of Bier's blocks in the ED, so please refer to this document for further information.

# Reference

https://www.rcem.ac.uk/docs/RCEM%20Guidance/Biers_block_revised_Nov_2017.pdf

## 4.13 **Sedation**

### Instructions for Candidate

Please consent the patient, then perform and teach the junior doctor about procedural sedation for manipulation of this patient's dislocated elbow.

### Mark Scheme Breakdown

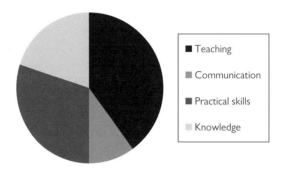

**Figure 4.13.1** Sedation mark scheme breakdown.

### Instructions for Actor

*Junior Doctor*

You are a Specialty Trainee Year 2 (ST2) doctor and you have a patient who has fallen off their bike and sustained an isolated dislocated elbow. You have never performed sedation or reduced an elbow before. You ask the candidate to explain conscious sedation and which drugs to use. You also ask how to assess an airway and which patients would not be suitable to sedate in the ED.

*Patient*

You have an isolated elbow injury. You are in a lot of pain and keen to have it fixed. You have not eaten or drunk anything for seven hours. You have never had an anaesthetic before. You have no health problems and take no medications. You have no known drug allergies. You have no loose teeth. There is a good range of movement of your neck. You understand the information provided to you and have no further questions.

### Instructions for Examiner

Observation only.

### Equipment Required

Full monitoring: pulse oximetry, cardiac monitoring, BP monitoring, end-tidal carbon dioxide ($ETCO_2$), IV access, fluids, sedation drugs.

# Mark Scheme

| | |
|---|---|
| Introduces self to patient and junior doctor | |
| Checks if the patient needs analgesia | |
| Establishes the ST2's previous experience and knowledge | |
| Asks if there are specific learning needs and sets learning objectives | |
| Obtains informed consent from the patient for sedation and manipulation: | |
| • Explains the benefits and risks, and the process | |
| • Invites questions and provides an information leaflet | |
| Asks permission to teach whilst performing the procedure | |
| Confirms dislocation on X-ray and checks the neurovascular status | |
| Assesses the patient: | |
| • Nil by mouth status | |
| • Asks about past medical history, drug history, allergies, weight, and past anaesthetic history | |
| • Performs an airway assessment (e.g. LEMON) and explains the components to the ST1 | |
| Sets up for procedure: | |
| • Ensures there is adequate staffing: two doctors and a nurse available | |
| • Ensures that full monitoring, resuscitation equipment, suction, airway trolley, $O_2$, emergency drugs, and plaster trolley are all available and checked | |
| • Considers preloading with fluids | |
| • Discusses appropriate choice of drugs (e.g. propofol 1% 1 mg/kg, ketamine 0.5–1 mg/kg) | |
| Performs set of observations | |
| Suggests using a safety checklist | |
| Discusses the endpoint of sedation: conscious sedation | |
| Teaches how to manipulate the elbow: | |
| • Applies inline traction, supinates the forearm to move the coronoid under the trochlea, and flexes the elbow whilst pushing directly on the tip of the olecranon | |
| Post-procedure care: | |
| • Observes until GCS 15, normal observations, no respiratory compromise or pain | |
| • Arranges and checks post-manipulation X-ray | |
| • Provides discharge advice and leaflet, and organises fracture clinic follow-up | |

| | |
|---|---|
| Invites questions from the patient and the ST1 | |
| Agrees a plan for ongoing learning with ST1 | |
| Suggests appropriate learning resources | |
| Good teaching style and rapport | |

Total    /**26**

## Learning Points

This is a difficult station as it can cover sedation, consent, and the procedure. It can be difficult to judge how much time to spend talking to the patient and how much time teaching. Be guided by the patient and the learning objectives stated by the student.

We suggest introducing yourself to both the patient and the student. Start by checking if the patient understands what the management plan entails and ask permission to teach. Then set the objectives with your student. Suggest teaching sedation/procedure and explain they can observe you consenting the patient and that you will talk about consent next time. Then quickly consent and move on to the rest of the task. LEMON airway assessment: Used to predict a difficult airway.

L: Look externally; facial hair, edentulous, sunken cheeks, obesity, facial trauma etc.

E: Evaluate using the 3-3-2 rule (3 finger breaths of mouth opening between incisors, 3 finger breaths hyoid-chin distance, 2 finger breaths for thyroid to floor of mouth).

M: Mallampati score: Above 2 suggests a more difficult airway.

O: Obstruction: Large tongue, trauma, quinsy/epiglottitis etc.

N: Neck mobility/range of movement.

## References

https://www.orthobullets.com/trauma/1018/elbow-dislocation
https://www.rcemlearning.co.uk/reference/adult-procedural-sedation/

# 4.14 Cervical Spine X-Ray Interpretation

## Instructions for Candidate

An F2 doctor has seen a patient following a low-speed car crash. She has assessed the patient and performed an X-ray but is not sure how to interpret it. Please go through the X-ray with her and answer any questions she has.

## Mark Scheme Breakdown

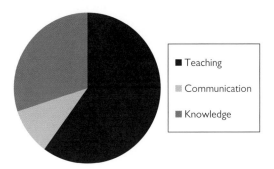

**Figure 4.14.1** Cervical spine X-ray interpretation mark scheme breakdown.

## Instructions for Actor

You are an F2 doctor with limited experience in the interpretation of cervical spine (C-spine) X-rays. You would like to be taught a system to interpret them. You are aware of the Canadian C-spine rules and believe your patient fits the rule for X-ray. The patient had a rear end shunt, was ambulatory on scene and in the ED, and now has delayed-onset midline C-spine tenderness, with no neurology.

## Instructions for Examiner

Observation only.

## Equipment Required

C-spine X-ray (Fig. 4.14.2).

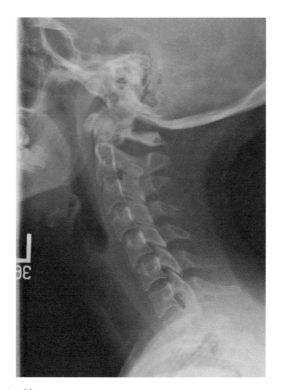

**Figure 4.14.2** C-spine X-ray.

From Fig 11.1 50 Imaging studies every doctor should know. Edited by Christoph I. Lee. Oxford University Press. ISBN 9780190223700.

## Mark Scheme

| | |
|---|---|
| Introduces self to junior doctor | |
| Establishes F2's previous experience and knowledge | |
| Asks if there are specific learning needs and sets learning objectives, e.g. focus on reviewing the lateral view X-ray today | |
| Confirms the history and mechanism, checks the patient is safe and requires no immediate treatment, and asks for examination findings | |
| Confirms the indications for the X-ray | |
| Talks through the X-ray interpretation: | |
| Confirms the patient's name, date, and time are correct | |
| Checks the adequacy from C1 to T1 | |
| Checks the alignment: | |

| | |
|---|---|
| • Anterior vertebral line | |
| • Posterior vertebral line | |
| • Posterior spinous process line | |
| Reviews each vertebral body contour, including the peg | |
| Reviews disc spaces | |
| Checks for soft tissue swelling | |
| Asks the F2 to review and talk through the patient's X-ray as taught | |
| Reinforces learning points and corrects any errors as necessary | |
| Formulates a management plan for the patient with a normal X-ray: | |
| • Examines the patient. If able to rotate head 45° left and right and has no midline tenderness and no neurological abnormalities, the patient can be discharged with analgesia and mobilisation advice | |
| Agrees a plan for ongoing learning: next session to cover anteroposterior (AP) and PEG views | |
| Suggests appropriate learning resources | |
| Is non-judgemental and facilitates learning | |

Total     **/19**

## Learning Points

*Prevertebral Soft Tissues*

Normal soft tissue parameters on the lateral view of a C-spine X-ray are:

- <7 mm at C2 and <22 mm at C6, or
- <50% of the vertebral body width above C4 and <100% of the vertebral body width below C4.

Widening of the soft tissue (i.e. due to a prevertebral haematoma) indicates a C-spine injury. However, normal parameters do not rule out injury, as not all C-spine fractures result in haematoma.

## Reference

https://www.radiologymasterclass.co.uk/tutorials/musculoskeletal/x-ray_trauma_spinal/x-ray_c-spine_normal

## 4.15 **Additional Stations**

The basic principles of a teaching station can be applied to virtually any skill, procedure, clinical scoring tool, or guideline. Remember that it need not involve the entire procedure and that you can select a particular section to be the focus of the teaching session, according to the student's learning needs. Use the generic mark schemes (see Sections 4.1 and 4.2) as a guide to develop your own stations. We have compiled an additional list of possible stations to help you:

- Eye examination/fundoscopy/discuss findings.
- Teaching any X-ray interpretation and management. Have a system for teaching CXR/pelvic X-ray (PXR)/abdominal X-ray (AXR)/spine X-ray and CT head.
- ECG interpretation: you cannot teach it all! Be selective; for example, describe the P wave, QRS complex, T wave, PR interval, and the rate and rhythm, and suggest that the next session will cover ST segments.
- GCS.
- Inhaler/spacer/peak flow technique.
- Non-invasive ventilation.
- Airway assessment and management.
- Teaching a guideline and discuss the management of the patient, e.g. NICE CT head, BTS pneumothorax.
- Gynaecological exam/speculum.
- Nerve blocks: femoral, fascia iliaca, wrist, ear.
- Rapid sequence induction of anaesthesia.
- Central line insertion.
- Arterial line insertion.
- Chest drain insertion.
- Joint aspiration.
- Lateral canthotomy.
- Catheter insertion.
- Cardioversion.

# Chapter 5 **Practical Skills and Procedures**

# The Practical Skills and Procedures Station

There will almost certainly be a practical procedure within the OSCE, possibly as part of a teaching station. Do not worry if you are not currently confident with the procedure itself—now is the time to practise so that by the time you sit the exam, you will be able to show the examiner how dexterous and skilled you are. Ensure that you know the indications for the procedure, as well as potential complications. Become familiar with the kit for each procedure, and practise handling it so that you do not fumble. Perform safety checks before starting. Review the patient on completion of the task.

For some of the more complex or time-consuming procedures, it is possible that you may be asked to perform just a section of it. For example, in a scenario requiring sedation and manipulation of a joint, you may be asked to obtain consent from the patient and perform an airway assessment, but then to simply talk through what drugs you would choose for the sedation or how you would per-form the reduction, rather than actually performing the skill. Of course, you should come to the exam prepared for any combination as you should be able to perform all the components of this scenario as a newly qualified consultant.

We really do urge you to practise the specific procedures, although there will be marks you can gain for simply completing several pre- and post-procedure actions that are generic to all stations. There will also be marks for communication and explanations to the patient, along with marks for the man-agement of the patient's condition and follow-up. We provide examples of generic mark schemes which you can adapt and use for any scenario.

# 5.1 **Generic Marks for Procedures**

It is sensible to break down a big task into smaller chunks. For a clinical procedure, this can be preparing for the procedure, obtaining consent, the actual procedure, and finally post-procedure care.

## Preparing for the Procedure

| | |
|---|---|
| Introduces self and confirms the patient's identity | |
| Washes hands | |
| Checks the patient is comfortable and offers analgesia | |
| Confirms the need for the procedure | |
| • Asks a brief, focused history | |
| • Requests to see relevant investigations, e.g. CXR, bladder scan, etc. | |
| • Confirms the side and site for the procedure | |

## Obtaining Informed Consent

| | |
|---|---|
| Discusses the indications for the procedure | |
| Explains the contraindications | |
| Explains the procedure | |
| Explains the potential complications | |
| Checks the patient's understanding and answers questions appropriately | |
| Provides an information leaflet to the patient | |

## Procedure

| | |
|---|---|
| Prepares the equipment/local anaesthetic/drugs for sedation | |
| Asks for a chaperone/assistant | |
| Washes hands, uses appropriate personal protective equipment | |
| Performs the procedure and explains each step as it is performed | |
| Disposes of sharps and used equipment | |

## Post-Procedure Care

| | |
|---|---|
| Offers to help the patient get dressed, ensures the patient is comfortable | |
| Discusses follow-up investigations, e.g. CXR to confirm chest drain position, or renal function following catheterisation | |
| Discusses follow-up care, e.g. wound care advice, tetanus immunisation, potential complications, fracture clinic | |
| Asks if there are any concerns or questions | |
| Ensures the procedure is recorded in the notes | |

Depending on how you use your time in the station, you may need to talk about the aftercare during the procedure, rather than once you have finished, e.g. discussing wound care and suture removal whilst placing the sutures.

## Examples of Practical Skills to Prepare

Some practical skills are more likely to be in the exam than others, but it is good practice to ensure you have prepared for them all. After all, the exam reflects what we do in real life.

- Airway assessment.
- Airway management.
- RSI.
- Procedural sedation.
- Setting up non-invasive ventilation.
- Insertion of chest drain.*
- Insertion of central line.
- Insertion of arterial line.
- IO access.
- Setting up a blood transfusion.
- Performing direct current (DC) cardioversion.
- Joint manipulation.
- Joint aspiration.
- Fracture manipulation.
- Suturing.
- Bier's block.
- Regional anaesthesia.**
- Urinary catheter insertion.
- Speculum PV examination.
- Fundoscopy.
- Otoscopy.
- Lateral canthotomy.

* Surgical and Seldinger.
** Femoral nerve block, fascia iliaca block, ankle block, auricular block, and wrist block.

## 5.2 **Catheterisation**

### Instructions for Candidate

A 65-year-old gentleman with previous curative treatment for bladder cancer has presented with severe lower abdominal pain, rosé-coloured urine, dysuria, and difficulty passing urine for 12 hours. Please assess and manage appropriately.

### Mark Scheme Breakdown

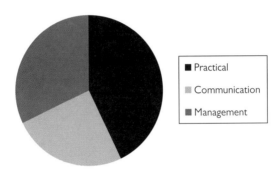

- ■ Practical
- ■ Communication
- ■ Management

**Figure 5.2.1** Catheterization mark scheme breakdown.

### Instructions for Actor

You are a 65-year-old gentleman with previous bladder cancer which was successfully treated with transurethral resection of bladder tumour (TURBT) and intravesical mitomycin. You have been suffering from pink urine for two days. It stings when you pass urine. You have been unable to pass urine all day and are in a lot of pain in your lower abdomen. You are nervous about having a catheter, as you previously had a bad experience, and you are very reluctant to have one and take some persuading. You are concerned the cancer has returned, as you had haematuria last time it was found. If the candidate does not mention follow-up management, ask if the cancer is back and what needs to happen now.

### Equipment Required

Catheter.
Instillagel.
Catheter pack.
Urometer.
Saline for cleaning.
Sterile gloves.

# Mark Scheme

| | |
|---|---|
| Introduces self and confirms the patient's identity | |
| Checks the patient is comfortable and offers analgesia | |
| Confirms the need for catheter (bladder scan/abdominal examination) | |
| Explains why the patient needs a catheter and addresses any concerns | |
| Obtains informed consent from the patient: | |
| • Discusses the indication, risk and benefits, complications, and alternatives | |
| Prepares the equipment | |
| Ensures there is privacy for the procedure | |
| Requests a chaperone | |
| Washes hands, uses sterile gloves (double layer) | |
| Exposes patient and covers with a sterile drape | |
| Cleans the penis | |
| Removes the outer gloves | |
| Inserts Instillagel and waits two minutes for it to become effective | |
| Places a kidney dish between the patient's legs to catch the urine | |
| With a non-touch technique, inserts the catheter | |
| Communicates with the patient throughout | |
| Ensures urine flowing and inflates the balloon | |
| Pulls the catheter back | |
| Connects the catheter to the catheter bag | |
| Gently returns the retracted foreskin to its normal position | |
| Disposes of waste | |
| Ensures the patient is comfortable and his dignity is maintained | |
| States will return to check the residual volume, take bloods (renal function), and dip the urine for signs of infection. State you will document in notes | |
| Explains the next steps to the patient: | |
| • The patient will need to be taught how to empty and change the bags | |
| • Await the blood test results today | |
| • Follow-up in the emergency urology clinic will be arranged | |
| Answers the patient's questions and addresses his concerns about cancer | |

Total    /28

## Learning Points

Practise this as a sterile technique at work until you can perform it skillfully and smoothly. Either use the two-glove technique or the clean hand/dirty hand technique, and do not cross-contaminate. Keeping the catheter in the plastic sleeve can be tricky to then feed into the urethra if you get lidocaine jelly everywhere, so practise!

## 5.3 **Fascia Iliaca Block**

### Instructions for Candidate

Please perform a fascia iliaca block (FIB) using the landmark technique on this patient with a left-sided fractured neck of femur.

### Mark Scheme Breakdown

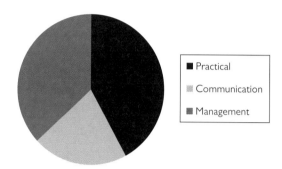

■ Practical

▨ Communication

■ Management

**Figure 5.3.1** Fascia iliaca block mark scheme breakdown.

### Instructions for Actor

You are a 76-year-old lady who slipped on icy ground and have fractured your left hip. You have had morphine and paracetamol in the ambulance, but your hip is still very painful. You have atrial fibrillation, and your international normalised ratio (INR) was checked yesterday and was 2.1; it has been stable for months. You have no known drug allergies. You weigh 66 kg.

### Instructions for Examiner

Ask the candidate to calculate the maximum dose of local anaesthetic that may be used, and confirm what dose they will use for this patient. Ask about contraindications if the candidate has not already mentioned them.

### Equipment Required

Dressing pack with sterile gloves.

0.5% chlorhexidine skin preparation.

Needles: a drawing-up needle, a 25 G (orange) needle, and a Tuohy needle or blunt nerve block needle.

Syringes: 2 ml, 2 × 20 ml, or 1 × 50 ml.

1% lidocaine.

0.25% bupivacaine.

# Mark Scheme

| | |
|---|---|
| Introduces self to the patient and confirms her identity | |
| Confirms the indication for the block | |
| Obtains consent: | |
| • Explains the indication, risks and benefits, complications, and alternatives | |
| Considers any contraindications, e.g. from past medical history, drug history, or allergies | |
| Checks the INR | |
| Checks and prepares the correct equipment | |
| Calculates the maximum local anaesthetic dose, draws up the appropriate volume of levobupivacaine | |
| Checks the X-ray and confirms the fracture and the site for the procedure | |
| Optimally positions the patient for the procedure | |
| Attaches the patient to monitoring and records the first set of observations—BP/ECG/O$_2$ saturations | |
| Identifies the landmarks [anterior superior iliac spine (ASIS), pubic tubercle, femoral pulse] and the insertion site | |
| Cleans and prepares the area | |
| Administers 1–2 ml of 1% lidocaine to the skin at the correct site | |
| Using the Tuohy needle, administers the correct dose of 0.25% levobupivacaine, aspirating and checking for blood every 5 ml | |
| Applies a dressing to the site | |
| Covers the patient to maintain dignity and ensures they are comfortable | |
| Checks the observations again and states will repeat them in 5, 10, 15, and 30 minutes | |
| Ensures the documentation and drug chart are completed | |
| Explains the next steps to the patient and invites questions | |

Total     /**19**

# Learning Points

FIB is a fairly common procedure to perform in emergency departments (EDs). The RCEM has published a guideline for FIB on its website, which is worth reading.

*Local Anaesthetic Choice*

A total volume of 1–2 ml of 1% lidocaine can be used for skin infiltration at the start of the procedure.

For FIB, 0.25% levobupivacaine is used. Use 30 ml if the patient weighs <50 kg or 40 ml if the patient weighs >50 kg. The maximum dose is 2 mg/kg.

*Landmarks*

The landmarks are the ASIS and pubic tubercle. Draw an imaginary line between the two, and then divide this line into thirds. The insertion point is 1 cm distal/caudal to the junction between the lateral 1/3 and medial 2/3s. The femoral pulse will, of course, be medial to this point.

*Procedure*

Using the Tuohy needle, pierce the skin. With the needle then in the sagittal plane, advance through two 'pops': the fascia lata and the fascia iliaca. Then advance the needle a further 1–2 mm. Aspirate to ensure the needle is not intravascular. Inject slowly, aspirating every 5 ml. Withdraw the needle, and apply gentle pressure to the area for up to two minutes.

Observations are recommended at 5, 10, 15, and 30 minutes, and then 4-hourly. Beware of patients who received opiates before the block and who may now suffer from their effects once the painful stimulus is removed. Ensure cardiac monitoring is attached.

*Complications*

Complications of FIB are failure, infection, bleeding, nerve damage, and local anaesthetic toxicity.

# References

https://www.rcem.ac.uk/docs/RCEM%20Guidance/Fascia_Iliaca_Block_in_the_Emergency_Department_ Revised_July_2020_v2.pdf

https://www.rcem.ac.uk/docs/Safety%20Resources%20+%20Guidance/Feb%20FIB%20Alert.pdf

## 5.4 **Seldinger Chest Drain Insertion**

### Instructions for Candidate

A 34-year-old male attended the ED, complaining of shortness of breath and pleuritic chest pain. An F2 doctor asks your advice regarding further management. The patient is haemodynamically stable. He has had a CXR (provided). Please explain the management to the patient and perform any necessary procedures.

### Mark Scheme Breakdown

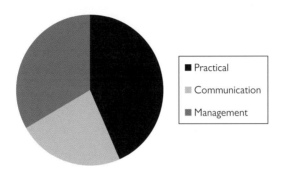

**Figure 5.4.1** Chest drain insertion mark scheme breakdown.

### Instructions for Actor

*F2 Doctor*

You have attempted to aspirate the pneumothorax and have taken another CXR which shows the pneumothorax is still >2 cm. You are uncertain of the next stage in this patient's management but are keen to aspirate again. You are not aware of the BTS guidelines and ask why the candidate is inserting a chest drain, rather than aspirating again.

You have not inserted a chest drain before. You would like to watch the candidate insert the chest drain and ask if the candidate could explain the steps as they happen. Ask the candidate to discuss further management.

*Patient*

You are 34 years old and present with your first spontaneous pneumothorax. You are a keen free diver, often diving to depths of 10 m unassisted. You are due to go on holiday to Bali next week for a week of free diving. If asked, volunteer this information and ask regarding future diving/flying. You are a non-smoker and do not have any medical problems. You become very upset when counselled regarding no further diving and not flying until fully resolved/followed up in the chest clinic. If the candidate does not show empathy, you become inconsolable and difficult and want a second opinion.

# Equipment Required

CXR (Fig. 5.4.2).
Seldinger chest drain kit.
Local anaesthetic.

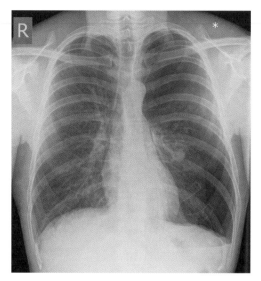

**Figure 5.4.2** Chest X-ray case 5.4.

# Mark Scheme

| | |
|---|---|
| Introduces self to the patient and confirms his identity | |
| Checks the patient is comfortable and offers him analgesia | |
| Confirms the need for the Seldinger chest drain | |
| Confirms the site from the CXR and chest auscultation | |
| Confirms the patient has normal clotting and platelets | |
| Explains the diagnosis and requirement for the chest drain | |
| Obtains informed consent from the patient: | |
| • Discusses the indication, the procedure, risk and benefits, complications, and alternatives | |
| Prepares and checks the equipment | |
| Ensures there is monitoring on, a cannula *in situ*, and an assistant is available | |

| | |
|---|---|
| Positions the patient sitting up, with the assistant supporting the patient's arm over his head | |
| Washes hands, puts on sterile gloves and gown, and covers the patient with a drape | |
| Correctly identifies the landmarks | |
| Uses local anaesthetic at the correct site | |
| Inserts the drain: | |
| • Inserts the needle, aspirates and confirms air in the pleural space | |
| • Threads the guidewire through needle | |
| • Makes a cut through the skin with the scalpel | |
| • Uses the dilators over the guidewire | |
| • Inserts the drain towards the apex at the appropriate length | |
| • Connects the drain to an underwater seal and ensures there is swinging | |
| • Sutures the drain and secures with a dressing | |
| • Disposes of sharps safely | |
| Ensures patient comfort and dignity are maintained | |
| Requests a post-procedure CXR | |
| Explains the follow-up to the patient: | |
| • Arranges admission until the lung has inflated and the drain can be removed | |
| • Arranges early review with the respiratory team | |
| Advises against flying for six weeks following resolution of the pneumothorax | |
| Sensitively advises that diving should be avoided permanently | |
| Advises against smoking and provides information about signs of recurrence | |
| Answers the patient's questions and addresses any concerns | |

Total    **/30**

## Learning Points

As with other procedures, practise the steps until there is fluency and dexterity to your movements. Familiarise yourself with the kit. Make use of simulation opportunities. Remember your communications skills—you are performing a procedure on a patient who may well be feeling anxious and in pain.

The management of a pneumothorax is discussed in Section 2.9 and Fig. 2.9.3.

# References

https://thorax.bmj.com/content/65/Suppl_2/ii18

https://thorax.bmj.com/content/thoraxjnl/57/4/289.full.pdf

https://www.caa.co.uk/Passengers/Before-you-fly/Am-I-fit-to-fly/Guidance-for-health-professionals/Respiratory-disease/

## 5.5  Airway Management and Intubation

### Instructions for Candidate

A 49-year-old lady has presented with a GCS of 6, having collapsed following a sudden onset of severe headache and vomiting. She has arrived in Resus with a supraglottic airway device *in situ*. Please manage this patient's airway and perform an RSI prior to transfer for a CT head.

### Mark Scheme Breakdown

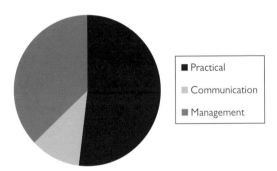

■ Practical

▨ Communication

■ Management

**Figure 5.5.1**  Airway management and intubation mark scheme breakdown.

### Instructions for Actor

*Nurse*

You are able to set up monitoring, insert cannulae, prepare arterial line sets, prepare drugs, perform cricoid pressure, and pass airway equipment appropriately. You can set up the ventilator if asked.

*Registrar*

You are a competent Specialty Trainee Year 3 (ST3), and you have completed a year of anaesthetics and intensive care training at ST2 level. You are able to assist in any way needed but do not wish to insert the endotracheal tube (ETT). Please ask the candidate for the doses of the drugs they are using.

When asked to call for senior help, explain everyone else is tied up with a trauma call but that the consultant is in the next bay and happy for you to carry on and will assist if there are any difficulties.

First intubation attempt: the candidate may think they have intubated the trachea, but please inform them there is no ETCO$_2$ trace, the chest is not rising, and there is no air entry. If they recognise the oesophageal intubation quickly and have a second attempt at intubation, you inform them that they were successful and O$_2$ saturations now remain >90%. If they fail to recognise the oesophageal intubation and do not attempt to reintubate, the patient will steadily deteriorate and eventually arrest.

## Equipment Required

Drugs.
ETTs.
Lubrication.
Laryngoscope.
Bougie.
Tie.
Ventilator.
Water circuit.
Intubation checklist (if asked for).

## Mark Scheme

| | |
|---|---|
| Introduces self to the team: states name and role | |
| Confirms the patient's GCS and the need for intubation | |
| Prepares for intubation: | |
| • Calls intensive therapy unit (ITU)/ED consultant for assistance | |
| • Sets up monitoring (ECG, BP, $O_2$ saturations, $ETCO_2$) | |
| • Ensures there are two sites of IV access | |
| • Prepares the appropriate drugs, including rescue medications | |
| • Pre-oxygenates the patient for two minutes | |
| • Optimises the patient's position for intubation | |
| • Allocates team roles (drug giver, airway assistant, cricoid) | |
| • Ensures IV fluids are given | |
| • Checks the equipment (suction, bag–valve–mask, ETT, lubrication, bougie, laryngoscopes) | |
| Discuss intubation plan A, B, and C | |
| Suggests completing the RSI checklist | |
| Proceeds with the intubation: | |
| • Gives appropriate doses of appropriate drugs | |
| • Ensures cricoid pressure is applied | |
| • Waits for fasciculation/one minute | |
| • Handles the laryngoscope and airway correctly | |

| | |
|---|---|
| • Inserts the tube | |
| • Confirms tube placement (chest movement, auscultation, ETCO$_2$) | |
| Recognises oesophageal intubation and removes the tube | |
| Has a second attempt at intubation (successful) | |
| Secures the tube and connects to the ventilator | |
| Asks for a long-acting muscle relaxant and appropriate maintenance infusion | |
| Mentions neuroprotective measures (tube tie not around the neck, 30° head up, BP control) | |
| Mentions completion of the transfer checklist prior to transfer to CT | |
| Answers questions and addresses any concerns appropriately | |
| Overall ensures a safe RSI and good team interaction and awareness | |

Total    /**27**

# Learning Points

The examiners do not have a specific formula for RSI drugs that you must use. Have a recipe in your head that you could use for most situations and mention doses if required, e.g. fentanyl 3 mcg/kg, ketamine 2 mg/kg and rocuronium 1 mg/kg, or propofol 2 mg/kg and suxamethonium 1.5 mg/kg or rocuronium. Remember to reduce the doses in the elderly or haemodynamically unstable patients. As long as you say something sensible, that is fine.

## 5.6 **Central Line Insertion**

### Instructions for Candidate

An 18-year-old student has presented with meningococcal sepsis. Please insert a central line prior to transfer to the ITU.

### Mark Scheme Breakdown

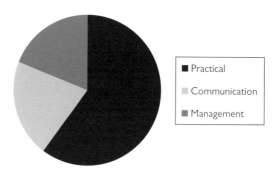

**Figure 5.6.1** Central line insertion mark scheme breakdown.

### Instructions for Actor

*Nurse*

You are an experienced resus nurse and able to help prepare the patient and equipment for this procedure when asked. The patient has deranged clotting, but the ITU is providing fresh frozen plasma (FFP)/appropriate blood products and is happy for you to proceed.

*Patient*

You are drowsy but understand what is going on. You will do whatever the candidate asks you and comply with the procedure if they explain what they are doing and talk to you as they go. If they are not reassuring and do not obtain consent appropriately, you will move around and contaminate the field.

### Equipment Required

Central line kit.
Local anaesthetic.
Sterile drapes, gown, gloves.

# Mark Scheme

| | |
|---|---|
| Introduces self to the patient and the team | |
| Checks the patient is comfortable and offers analgesia | |
| Confirms the need for a central line | |
| Explains to the patient in a reassuring manner what a central line is and why it is needed | |
| Obtains informed consent from the patient: | |
| • Discusses the indication, risks and benefits, complications, and alternatives | |
| Prepares the equipment, e.g. local anaesthetic, ultrasound machine, procedure trolley | |
| Sets up monitoring (ECG, BP, O$_2$ saturations) | |
| Ensures there are two sites of IV access | |
| Positions the patient 10° head down and head turned laterally | |
| Identifies landmarks correctly | |
| Mentions will perform the procedure under ultrasound guidance | |
| Scrubs up, puts on sterile gown and gloves, uses a sterile probe cover | |
| Exposes the patient, cleans the skin, and covers the patient with a sterile drape | |
| Infiltrates with local anaesthetic | |
| Prepares the central line catheter, flushes and closes the line and all the connectors | |
| Demonstrates a good view with the USS and correctly identifies the internal jugular vein (IJV) and carotid artery | |
| Inserts the introducer needle at 30° to skin, aiming towards the ipsilateral nipple and aspirating until flashback seen and the needle visualised on the USS to enter the IJV | |
| Disconnects the needle, inserts the guidewire to the 10 cm mark, removes the needle | |
| Makes a small incision in the skin and uses the dilators in series | |
| Inserts the catheter over the wire, maintaining contact with wire. Inserts to 12–15 cm, aiming the tip of the catheter at the carina | |
| Puts the connector on the catheter and aspirates, and then flushes the line | |
| Secures the catheter with sutures and a dressing | |
| Maintains a sterile field and situational awareness with the patient | |
| Disposes of sharps safely | |

| Confirms the patient is comfortable | |
|---|---|
| Requests a post-procedure CXR and ensures the documentation is complete | |
| Explains the next steps to the patient and addresses any concerns | |
| Good communication with patient throughout procedure | |

Total    /**28**

# Learning Points

This station provides another opportunity for you to demonstrate your ability to perform a complex task. A significant portion of the marks is given for appropriate preparation—both of the patient and of the equipment, as well as post-procedure care, so ensure these actions are part of your routine practice.

The landmarks for central line insertion are shown in Fig. 5.6.2.

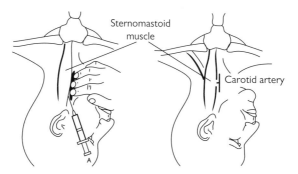

**Figure 5.6.2** Internal jugular cannulation.

Reproduced with permission from *https://oxfordmedicine.com/view/10.1093/med/9780198784197.001.0001/ med-9780198784197-chapter-2#med-9780198784197-chapter-2-div1-39*

## 5.7 **Condom Retrieval**

### Instructions for Candidate

A 19-year-old girl attends at 3 am, upset. She was having sex with a new partner and the condom came off. She believes the condom is still PV. Please remove the condom, assess her risk of STIs, and counsel as appropriate.

### Mark Scheme Breakdown

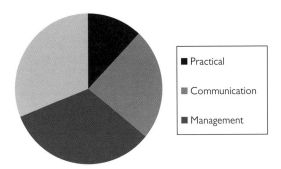

- ■ Practical
- ■ Communication
- ■ Management

**Figure 5.7.1** Condom retrieval mark scheme breakdown.

### Instructions for Actor

You are a 19-year-old student. You had sex for the first time with a new casual partner tonight. You know nothing about his sexual health. You have had three sexual partners since starting university four weeks ago. You used condoms with them all and you are on the oral contraceptive pill (OCP). You have not missed any pills. You have only ever had vaginal sex and have given unprotected oral sex. You have never had a sexual health screen. Your LMP was three weeks ago. You have not had any discharge or pain. You had a long-term boyfriend back home before starting university, but that ended as your boyfriend cheated on you. You have never had sex with a sex worker or anyone from a high-risk area.

You answer all questions truthfully, although you feel very awkward. You are shocked if the doctor suggests a sexual health check but are keen once it is explained to you. You ask if it is OK to wait until the genitourinary medicine (GUM) clinic review before receiving antibiotics, as you are keen to start them now if you are at risk of STIs.

### Equipment Required

Speculum.
Lubrication.
Magill forceps.

Sheet.
Bed.
Tissues.
Gloves.

## Mark Scheme

| | |
|---|---|
| Introduces self to the patient | |
| Checks the patient is comfortable and offers analgesia | |
| Clarifies the history of the presenting complaint | |
| Asks about past medical history and drug and social history, including drugs and alcohol | |
| Explains that you would like to perform bimanual/speculum to remove condom | |
| Suggests discussing sexual health after the procedure | |
| Explains the procedure | |
| Arranges a chaperone to be present | |
| Ensures privacy for the procedure and allows the patient to undress in privacy | |
| Performs the examination: | |
| • Inspects | |
| • Performs bimanual palpation | |
| • Uses the speculum and retrieves the condom | |
| • Re-examines to confirm no other foreign bodies or abnormalities | |
| • Ensures the patient is comfortable and offers privacy to dress | |
| Communicates and reassures appropriately during the procedure | |
| Disposes of waste | |
| Sensitively takes a sexual history: | |
| • Asks about this incident: partner/type of sex/consensual/confirm OCP (missed pills, where in pack) | |
| • Asks about other partners: how many/casual or regular partners/sex of partners/type of sex/protected/concerns about STIs | |
| • Asks about her usual contraception | |
| • Asks about sex with high-risk partners: sex workers/known bloodborne virus/STIs/ from high-risk countries | |
| • Asks about previous sexual health checks, STIs, and treatment | |

| | |
|---|---|
| • Asks about discharge or pain PV or abdominal | |
| • Asks about periods: LMP/regularity/irregular bleeding | |
| Asks if there are any specific concerns | |
| Explains that if there were no missed pills, emergency contraception is not needed | |
| Advises the patient not to miss any pills in the next week | |
| Advises GUM clinic review tomorrow and gives contact details/drop-in clinic times, and explains the importance of a sexual health review | |
| Advises a blood test now for BBVs, with further tests and follow-up in the GUM clinic | |
| Discusses the need for PEP: low-risk partner, so no need for PEP (receiving vaginal sex carries a risk of <0.1%; 0.02% with oral sex) | |
| Advises hepatitis B vaccine | |
| Advises a pregnancy test now, and repeat if the next period is late | |
| Explains that the GUM team will screen for STIs and prescribe antibiotics if necessary | |
| Answers the patient's questions and addresses any concerns | |

Total    /**33**

# Learning Points

This station is tricky as there is a lot of history to get through, as well as an examination and a discussion of ongoing management. Practise taking a full sexual history at work; be confident in asking the relevant questions, and do not be embarrassed—just have a bank of questions that are standard in all cases. Be prepared to do the examination whilst discussing ongoing management if needed, to complete the task on time.

As always, be familiar with the equipment that you will use. The patient will be feeling vulnerable, so sensitive communication is a must. The rules for missed contraceptive pills and options for emergency contraception are outlined in the learning points of Section 2.6. The use of PEP is discussed in Section 2.13.

## 5.8 **Ear Laceration Requiring Field Block**

### Instructions for Candidate

Please insert a regional block and suture this patient's ear.

### Mark Scheme Breakdown

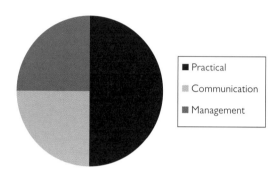

**Figure 5.8.1** Ear laceration requiring field block mark scheme breakdown.

### Instructions for Actor

You are a 20-year-old judo enthusiast. You have presented to the ED with a laceration to your earlobe. It happened during a judo competition today. You now have a very painful earlobe and will not allow the candidate to touch it. If the candidate suggests injecting local anaesthetic into your earlobe, you refuse to let them touch it as it is too painful. You will allow them to put a block in once they have explained where the injection goes.

### Equipment Required

Local anaesthetic.
Needle and syringe.
Suture kit.
Dressing.

### Mark Scheme

| | |
|---|---|
| Introduces self and confirms the patient's identity | |
| Checks the patient is comfortable and offers analgesia | |
| Confirms the need for suturing of laceration | |
| Obtains informed consent from the patient: | |

| | |
|---|---|
| • Discusses the indications, risk and benefits, complications, and alternatives | |
| Prepares the equipment | |
| Washes hands, puts on sterile gloves | |
| Infiltrates 10 ml of lidocaine 1% to achieve a field block | |
| Confirms the block is successful | |
| Cleans the skin | |
| Sutures the laceration | |
| Applies a dressing to the ear and gives follow-up wound care advice | |
| Disposes of sharps safely | |
| Ensures the patient is comfortable | |
| Advises the patient to keep the ear clean and dry and to avoid contact sports until resolved | |
| Answers the patient's questions and addresses his concerns | |

Total    /**20**

## Learning Points

*Performing a Field Block*

Use 10 ml of 1% lidocaine and infiltrate at points 1 and 2.

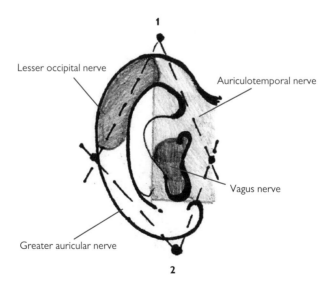

**Figure 5.8.2** Landmarks for a field block of the ear.

Point 1 (Fig. 5.8.2) is 1 cm below the lobe. Aim the needle anteriorly to the tragus, and then withdraw and aim posteriorly along the posterior surface in the skin crease. This provides the greater auricular nerve block.

Point 2 (Fig. 5.8.2) is where the helix meets the scalp. Aim the needle anteriorly to the tragus to gain an auriculotemporal block, then withdraw and aim posteriorly to the ear to achieve a lesser occipital nerve block.

### General Points Regarding Nerve Blocks

It is possible you could be asked to perform or teach a variety of nerve blocks. Consider revising the anatomy and technique for wrist, digital, supraorbital, ankle, and femoral nerve blocks.

Below is a generic mark scheme that can be applied to any nerve block.

| | |
|---|---|
| Introduces self and confirms the patient's identity | |
| Checks the patient is comfortable and offers analgesia | |
| Confirms the need for the procedure | |
| Obtains informed consent from the patient: | |
| • Discusses the indications | |
| • Considers any contraindications to the block (refusal, anticoagulation, infection at site, local anaesthetic allergy, femoral nerve bypass surgery at site) | |
| • Explains the procedure | |
| • Discusses risks and benefits | |
| • Discusses complications (intravascular injection, nerve damage, bleeding, infection, allergy/toxicity, pain, failure to work) | |
| • Discusses alternatives to the procedure, e.g. local anaesthetic, haematoma block, Bier's block, sedation, general anaesthesia | |
| Prepares the equipment and calculates the dose of local anaesthetic (possible question on max doses) | |
| Washes hands, puts on gloves | |
| Cleans the skin | |
| Considers the use of USS | |
| Safely introduces the local anaesthetic | |
| Safely disposes of sharps | |
| Checks the adequacy of the block | |
| Ensures the procedure is documented in the notes | |
| Confirms the patient is comfortable | |
| Explains the next steps to patient | |
| Answers the patient's questions and addresses any concerns | |

## 5.9 **Sedation and DC Cardioversion**

### Instructions for Candidate

A 45-year-old lady presents with clear onset of palpitations two hours ago and feeling light-headed on standing. She feels uncomfortable and has some chest pain. She has had an ECG. She had no previous episodes. Please manage this patient.

### Mark Scheme Breakdown

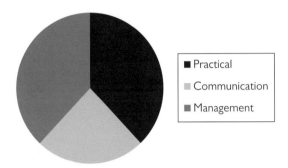

**Figure 5.9.1** Sedation and DC cardioversion mark scheme breakdown.

### Instructions for Actor

You are a 45-year-old lady with a first episode of arrhythmia. You are otherwise fit and well, take no medications, and have no allergies. This started ten minutes after you woke up, so you have not yet had anything to eat or drink today. You have no history of past anaesthetic problems.

You have some chest pain, and you are light-headed on standing. You are anxious to resolve the issue. If given the choice of electrical or chemical cardioversion, you opt for electrical. If only offered chemical, you ask if there are any alternatives and steer the scenario towards electrical cardioversion.

### Equipment Required

Defibrillator.
Monitored Resus bed with resuscitation equipment.
Sedation drugs.
ECG (Fig. 5.9.2).

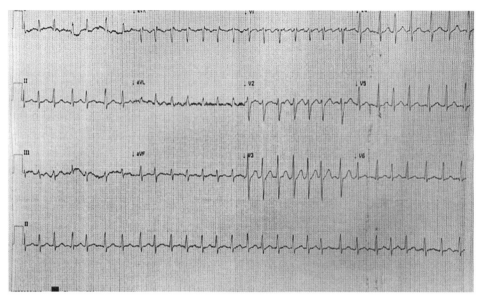

**Figure 5.9.2** ECG case 5.9.

## Reference

https://oxfordmedicine.com/view/10.1093/med/9780199654901.001.0001/med-9780199654901-chapter-8?rskey= 77yi4P&result=9

## Mark Scheme

| Introduces self to the patient and the nurse | |
|---|---|
| Confirms atrial fibrillation (AF) with rapid ventricular rate on the ECG | |
| Confirms the time of onset of symptoms and that this is the first episode | |
| Asks about past medical history, drug history, and allergies | |
| Explains the diagnosis to the patient | |
| Obtains informed consent from the patient for sedation and DC cardioversion: | |
| • Explains the intended procedure | |
| • Explains the alternatives: chemical cardioversion | |
| • Discusses the risks and benefits | |
| • Discusses possible complications | |
| Confirms the patient's anaesthetic history: | |
| • Asks about her fasting status | |

| | |
|---|---|
| • Asks about any previous anaesthetic problems | |
| • Assesses the airway (LEMON) | |
| • Weighs the patient | |
| Prepares for the procedure: | |
| • Ensures two doctors and a nurse are available | |
| • Ensures full monitoring, resuscitation equipment, suction, airway trolley, $O_2$, emergency drugs, and plaster trolley are available and checked | |
| • Selects appropriate drugs for the sedation, e.g. propofol 1% 1 mg/kg, ketamine 0.5–1 mg/kg | |
| • Considers preloading with fluids | |
| • Turns the defibrillator on, sets it to synchronised mode, and selects the energy level (120–150 J) | |
| Suggests using a checklist and performs a set of observations | |
| Discuss the endpoint of sedation: conscious sedation | |
| Delivers a synchronised DC shock | |
| Confirms the rhythm, repeats the shock if necessary | |
| Post-procedure care: | |
| • Observes the patient until her GCS is 15 and she has normal observations and no respiratory compromise or any pain | |
| • Reviews the post-cardioversion ECG | |
| • Advises follow up with cardiology | |
| Answers the patient's questions and addresses any concerns | |

Total    /**27**

## Learning Points

This is a very extensive scenario with several components that could be tested in the exam. The actual delivery of the DC shock only gains 1 point. The bulk of the mark scheme is associated with the preparation, so you must demonstrate to the examiner that you have assessed the patient, the procedure is indicated, and you have performed adequate safety and equipment checks. After the cardioversion, demonstrate appropriate post-procedure care. We have included the whole scenario with marks for consent, sedation, and procedure for completeness.

It is possible that you may be asked to perform just a part of this scenario. For example, the focus could be on consent, sedation, or the cardioversion itself. We have provided all elements here for completeness, but we suspect this may be more than you would be expected to do in one station (see LEMON, Chapter 4).

## 5.10 **Lateral Canthotomy**

### Instructions for Candidate

A 44-year-old cricket player has taken a direct blow to his right eye. He is complaining of pain in the eye and has reduced movement and visual acuity. On examination, there is proptosis of the eye, with a relative afferent pupillary defect and a raised intraocular pressure >40 mmHg. Please manage this patient's condition.

### Mark Scheme Breakdown

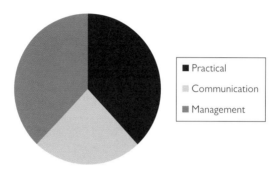

**Figure 5.10.1** Lateral canthotomy mark scheme breakdown.

### Instructions for Actor

You are a 44-year-old teacher, and you were playing cricket with your A-level students when you received a blow with the ball to your right eye. You are now in a lot of pain, can only see a blur, and cannot move your eye properly.

### Instructions for Examiner

Inform candidate there are no signs of globe rupture if asked.

### Equipment Required

Scalpel.
1% lidocaine and syringe.
Clamp.

# Mark Scheme

| | |
|---|---|
| Introduces self to the patient | |
| Offers the patient analgesia | |
| Explains the diagnosis to the patient (retrobulbar haemorrhage) | |
| Explains the required procedure (lateral canthotomy) | |
| Requests an urgent ophthalmology review (unavailable) | |
| Obtains informed consent from the patient: | |
| • Discusses the indications, risks and benefits, complications, and alternatives | |
| Mentions contraindication: globe rupture (informed examined and not ruptured) | |
| Prepares the equipment | |
| Considers sedation | |
| Washes hands, puts on sterile gloves | |
| Cleans the skin around the eye | |
| Infiltrates 1–2 ml of 1% lidocaine with adrenaline into the lateral canthus, aiming away from the globe | |
| Devascularises the lateral canthus with a clamp for one minute | |
| Cuts the lateral canthus, then cuts the inferior and lateral tendons | |
| Rechecks the intraocular pressure | |
| Advises acetazolamide and timolol eye drops | |
| Ensures an urgent ophthalmology review | |
| Explains the follow-up to the patient if he is awake | |
| Answers the patient's questions and addresses any concerns | |

Total    **/21**

# Learning Points

An emergency lateral canthotomy following trauma to the eye is not a common procedure, but when it is required, it needs to be done promptly and efficiently. The mark scheme demonstrates that even if you are not 100% familiar with performing the procedure, you could still score many of the marks for good pre-procedure and post-procedure care. Make a sensible attempt at the procedure itself, as even if done incorrectly, you would only lose a couple of marks.

Simple search terms, such as 'lateral canthotomy', will generate articles, tutorials, and videos online. EM:RAP and East Midlands Emergency Medicine Educational Media are two useful sources. To our knowledge, this station has not come up in previous sittings of the OSCE, but it is useful to be prepared for unusual stations. It is also very worthwhile being prepared to perform a lateral canthotomy in real life.

# References

EM:RAP. *How to do a lateral canthotomy*. https://www.youtube.com/watch?v=tgQaKVGynFA
EM3 Resus Drills. *Lateral canthotomy*. https://em3.org.uk/foamed/31/1/2020/resus-drills-lateral-canthotomy

# Chapter 6 **Communication**

# The Communication Station

Communication is a strong focus in many types of OSCE stations. There will be marks in any patient-focused station such as history and management, breaking bad news, or explaining a diagnosis. There will be elements in any station where liaison with colleagues is involved. Remember to stay calm and non-confrontational at all times, be the patient's advocate, and explain things clearly when asked. You need to establish a good rapport in the patient-centred consultation, even if you need to be firm such as in a non-accidental injury (NAI) or a difficult patient station. Although advanced communication skills or dealing with conflict may not come naturally to some, with practice, you can score highly on these stations.

## 6.1 **Requesting Antibiotics**

### Instructions for Candidate

Please take a brief history and perform a focused examination for this one-year-old boy called Tom. He presented with his mum with a two-day history of fever and a sore ear. Please explain the diagnosis and management to his mum.

### Mark Scheme Breakdown

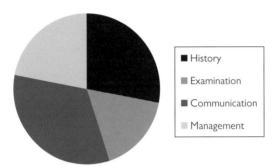

- ■ History
- ■ Examination
- ■ Communication
- ■ Management

**Figure 6.1.1** Requesting antibiotics mark scheme breakdown.

### Instructions for Actor

You are a very anxious, well-educated mother of one-year-old Tom. You are very concerned that he has an ear infection and needs antibiotics. He has had a fever and was tugging on his right ear. You gave him some paracetamol this morning, which has brought the temperature down. His oral intake this morning was minimal, but he has managed some lunch and has had a snack in the waiting room. You are very insistent he should have antibiotics as he clearly has an infection. If the candidate offers you a sound explanation of why he does not require them, you will calm down and accept the explanation. If, however, they fail to explain adequately why not, then you become angry and will ask for a second opinion.

### Instructions for Examiner

When the candidate asks to examine the patient, please provide any examination findings they ask for:

Well hydrated, CRT <2 seconds.

Chest is clear on auscultation.

Inflamed and bulging tympanic membrane on the right side.

Tonsils are normal.

No lymphadenopathy.

Afebrile, observations are normal.

# Equipment Required

Torch and tongue depressor.
Otoscope.

# Mark Scheme

| | |
|---|---|
| Introduces self to the patient and his mother | |
| Offers analgesia | |
| Takes a focused history: | |
| • Asks about the presenting complaint | |
| • Asks for more details, e.g. onset, pain, which ear affected, discharge from the ear | |
| • Asks about associated symptoms, e.g. fever, cough, rash, level of alertness | |
| • Asks about fluid intake and output | |
| Past medical history | |
| Drug history (including immunisations) and allergies | |
| Examines the child: | |
| • Asks to see observations chart | |
| • Comments on hydration status | |
| • Feels for lymphadenopathy | |
| • Examines the throat | |
| • Examines the ears | |
| • Auscultates the chest | |
| • Demonstrates a good rapport with the child | |
| Explains the diagnosis of acute otitis media | |
| Explains that most cases are viral and get better without antibiotics | |
| Explains that in this case, there is no need for antibiotics | |
| Explains the treatment is analgesia, oral fluids, and supportive treatment | |
| Answers mum's questions and addresses her concerns | |
| Explains the risks of taking unnecessary antibiotics | |
| Sensitively negotiates and agrees on a plan with mum (either no antibiotics or a delayed backup prescription) | |

| | |
|---|---|
| Demonstrates a non-confrontational manner and successfully reassures the mother | |
| Discharges the patient with a safety net to return if symptoms worsen rapidly or significantly, or patient becomes unwell | |

Total    /**24**

# Learning Points

Acute otitis media (AOM) is a common diagnosis and parents sometimes think that antibiotics are indicated. This station gives you the opportunity to show your knowledge of the NICE guidelines and discuss with the parent when it is appropriate to prescribe antibiotics for the child.

Without antibiotic treatment, 60% of patients get better in 24 hours and 80% in three days, although symptoms can last up to one week. Antibiotics should be offered in AOM if the child:

- Is systemically very unwell.
- Has significant comorbidities or has high risk of complications.
- Has had symptoms for >3 days without improvement.

Children with AOM are more likely to benefit from antibiotics if the child:

- Is under two years old and has bilateral infection.
- Has otorrhoea.

First-line treatment is with amoxicillin for five to seven days.

# Reference

https://www.nice.org.uk/guidance/ng91/resources/visual-summary-pdf-4787282702

## 6.2 **Child Maltreatment**

### Instructions for Candidate

Peter has been sent for an X-ray of his leg from triage. He is 18 months old. Mum has brought him in as he has not been weight-bearing on his left leg for three days. Please review Peter and the X-ray, and explain the management to his mother.

### Mark Scheme Breakdown

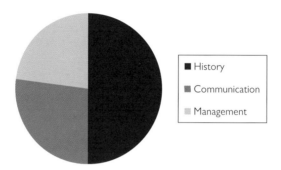

**Figure 6.2.1** Child maltreatment mark scheme breakdown.

### Instructions for Actor

You are the mother of Peter. He is a loud and boisterous 18-month old. You live alone and have no support. You noticed Peter limping a few days ago and now he is not walking on his left leg. You do not know how he sustained the injury. If pressed on this, you will later change your story and say he fell down some steps a few days ago. You become very defensive and angry, and feel you are being blamed for the injury. When the doctor advises admitting Peter for further investigation, you begin to cry and shout and say that you are leaving. When the doctor explains the gravity of the situation and that the police will be involved if you leave, you sit down and agree to stay.

### Instructions for Examiner

If the candidate removes Peter's clothes for the examination, state that there are fingertip-shaped bruises visible around Peter's chest.

### Equipment Required

X-ray leg: metaphyseal corner fracture/bucket handle fracture (Fig. 6.2.2).

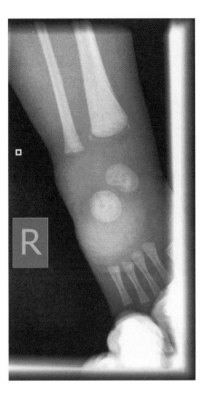

**Figure 6.2.2** X-ray leg.

Reproduced from fig 14.10.16 Tibial and ankle fractures in children. Oxford Textbook of Trauma and Orthopaedics (2nd Edition) by Christopher Bulstrode, James Wilson-MacDonald, Deborah M. Eastwood, John McMaster, Jeremy Fairbank, Parminder J. Singh, Sandeep Bawa et al. Oxford University Press. ISBN 9780199550647.

## Mark Scheme

| | |
|---|---|
| Introduces self to Peter and his mum, and confirms their identity and relationship | |
| Offers analgesia | |
| Uses an open question to ask about the presenting complaint | |
| Establishes the details: | |
| • Asks what happened and when. Asks when the limp was first noticed | |
| • Asks who was with the child at the time of the injury | |
| • Clarifies why there has been a delay in presentation | |
| Clarifies Peter's motor development and correlates this with the history given | |
| Asks about previous ED attendances or injuries | |

| | |
|---|---|
| Past medical history (including perinatal problems) | |
| Drug history (including immunisations) and allergies | |
| Social history, including family structure | |
| Asks about childcare settings and who else looks after Peter | |
| Asks about any contact with social services or the health visitor | |
| Asks to examine Peter | |
| Fully undresses Peter to examine him from head to toe | |
| Carefully inspects Peter and looks specifically for bruises and injuries | |
| Explains that the X-ray reveals a fracture and that Peter will need a plaster cast | |
| Explains that the type of injury sustained and the delayed presentation are causes for concern | |
| Explains that Peter will be referred to the paediatric team for further review in hospital | |
| Explains that further examination and investigations may be needed | |
| Informs the need to discuss the case with social services | |
| Explains that if mum tries to leave with Peter, the police will be involved to ensure his welfare | |
| Establishes a rapport with mother and is firm, but not accusatory | |
| Reassures mum that Peter's welfare and well-being are the greatest priority | |
| Answers final questions and addresses any remaining concerns | |

Total      /**25**

# Learning Points

This station may initially look like a straightforward minor injuries case. This would be unusual for the FRCEM, so expect another element. Note the distribution of marks from the pie chart. If you take a thorough history, specifically obtaining details of the mechanism, and take cues from the mother's body language, you will quickly realise this is not straightforward. Always remember the additional elements of social history for children as this again may alert you to NAI and will be on the mark scheme.

Children may present with seemingly small injuries, but we must remain vigilant to the possibility of NAI. Do not be scared to ask further questions if the mechanism described is inconsistent with the injury sustained or the age of the child. If there is a delayed presentation, or the story changes be suspicious.

The following injuries should raise suspicion:

- Bruising: in non-mobile babies, in unusual sites such as the medial aspect of the thighs and upper arms; bruises suspicious for finger or object imprinting or bite marks.

- Fractures: multiple, especially if of varying ages; in non-mobile children; rib and spine fractures; long bone fractures in children <3 years.
- Fractures associated with rotation, shaking, and pulling, as in this scenario, including epiphyseal separation and metaphyseal fractures of the knee, wrist, elbow, and ankle.
- Torn frenulum.
- Genital injuries.
- Burns to the buttocks/lower limbs suggesting hot water immersion.
- Round burns suggestive of cigarette burns.

Observe the child's emotional status, body language, and interaction with parents. If there is any concern, discuss with the paediatric or safeguarding consultant.

There is a useful module on *Radiopedia* complete with images suspicious for NAI (see References below).

# References

https://oxfordmedicine.com/view/10.1093/med/9780198784197.001.0001/med-9780198784197-chapter-15# med-9780198784197-chapter-15-div1-530

https://radiopaedia.org/articles/suspected-physical-abuse-1

## 6.3 **Blood Transfusion Refusal**

### Instructions for Candidate

You have assessed 66-year-old Jim in Resus and have found him to have a ruptured spleen, having fallen off his bike today. His haemoglobin is 55 g/l and he is shocked. Your surgical colleagues have assessed him and are preparing to take him to theatre imminently. They have asked you to resuscitate and stabilise with blood products in the meantime.

Jim is a devout Jehovah's Witness and is refusing blood products. Please talk to the patient and agree a plan.

### Mark Scheme Breakdown

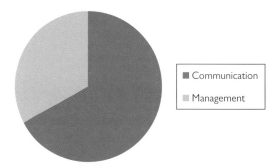

**Figure 6.3.1** Blood transfusion refusal mark scheme breakdown.

### Instructions for Actor

You are a 66-year-old Jehovah's Witness. You are strongly against blood products and refuse to accept them. You have full capacity. You understand that you may die without a transfusion and are willing to take this risk.

You will accept surgery, and if offered, you will consider cell salvage and tranexamic acid.

### Instructions for Examiner

Observation only.

### Equipment Required

None.

## Mark Scheme

| | |
|---|---|
| Introduces self to the patient | |
| Checks the patient is aware of the CT results and explains what it means | |
| Explains that surgery is required to control the bleeding | |
| Explains the blood loss is significant and that the treatment includes a blood transfusion and emergency surgery | |
| Listens to the patient's concerns and the patient wishes to not receive blood products | |
| Explains the potential consequences of not receiving a blood transfusion, which includes death | |
| Checks the patient's understanding of what has been discussed | |
| Discusses other options, e.g. cell salvage, fluids, erythropoietin (EPO) | |
| Asks the patient to demonstrate they can retain the information given | |
| Checks the patient can weigh up the risks and benefits | |
| Confirms the patient can communicate their wishes | |
| Allows the patient to explain his decision | |
| Offers the patient the opportunity to speak to a trusted advocate, e.g. next of kin | |
| Offers the patient some time to consider the information before making a final decision | |
| Confirms there has been no coercion in the decision to refuse blood | |
| Ensures the team is aware of the decision and that the discussion is documented in the patient's notes | |
| Reassures the patient that he will not be discriminated against because of his decision | |
| Explains the next steps in the management: | |
| • Ongoing treatment with tranexamic acid and fluids | |
| • Preparation for transfer to theatre | |
| Demonstrates a non-judgemental attitude | |

Total    **/20**

## Learning Points

Competent adults can refuse treatment with blood products, even if it seems irrational and can result in death. However, in an emergency, if doubt exists regarding capacity or the validity of a blood refusal card, aim to preserve life and give the necessary blood.

*Parental Refusal of Treatment for a Child*

Parents cannot refuse blood for their children in a life-threatening situation. This is based on:

- The child's best interests are those of the state and outweigh the parental rights to refuse medical treatment.
- Parental rights do not give the parents life and death authority over their children.
- Parents do not have an absolute right to refuse medical treatment based on religious beliefs if the refusal is regarded as unreasonable.

# Reference

https://www.gmc-uk.org/ethical-guidance/ethical-guidance-for-doctors/personal-beliefs-and-medical-practice/personal-beliefs-and-medical-practice

## 6.4 Breaking Bad News

### Instructions for Candidate

A 56-year-old man called Mr Jenkins was brought in by ambulance in cardiac arrest. He had 45 minutes of cardiopulmonary resuscitation (CPR) prehospital and arrived in asystole. You continued to resuscitate and performed a blood gas and an echocardiography, and the decision was taken to cease the resuscitation.

His wife has just arrived and is in the relative's room. She was not on scene with him and only knows that he collapsed whilst out shopping. Please inform Mrs Jenkins about what has happened.

### Mark Scheme Breakdown

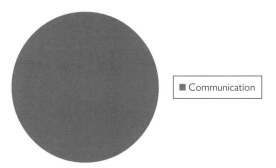

**Figure 6.4.1** Breaking bad news mark scheme breakdown.

### Instructions for Actor

You are Mrs Jenkins. You have been married for 36 years. You are here with your son. You were brought in by the police as they were notified that your husband had collapsed in the supermarket. You do not know that he has suffered a cardiac arrest.

You are distraught and cry and scream when told the news. You cannot believe what has happened. You knew he had high BP and was a bit overweight, but he has been well this week. He had complained of chest pain whilst out walking a few days before and does get a bit out of breath climbing the stairs, but he has not seen his GP. When you have calmed down, you ask about organ donation as you are sure this is what he would have wanted, although you are worried as you do not want them to take his eyes.

### Instructions for Examiner

Observation only.

# Equipment Required

None.

# Mark Scheme

| | |
|---|---|
| Introduces self to the patient | |
| Confirms their names and relationship to the patient | |
| Asks if they would like anyone else present | |
| Acknowledges the difficult and unexpected circumstances | |
| Clarifies their knowledge of events so far | |
| Sensitively provides a brief background of events leading to the present | |
| Sensitively breaks the bad news, avoiding the use of jargon or euphemisms | |
| Makes good use of silence and timing and does not rush the conversation | |
| Offers sincere condolences | |
| Offers to provide further explanations and details | |
| Offers to contact a friend or relative or chaplain for support | |
| Provides a bereavement leaflet and explains the bereavement process | |
| Offers the opportunity to see the patient | |
| Briefs the relatives on what to expect when seeing the patient | |
| Reassures you will be available to see them again after they have seen their relative | |
| Invites questions about the discussion so far | |
| Answers Mrs Jenkins' questions regarding organ donation: | |
| • Explains that the organ donation team will speak to her and give more information | |
| • Reassures Mrs Jenkins that the team will address her ideas, concerns, and expectations regarding organ donation | |
| • Explains that after donation, the body would be returned to the family to make funeral arrangements | |
| Answers any further questions | |
| Takes the family to see Mr Jenkins | |

| Establishes a good rapport with the family, is empathetic, and conveys important information | |
| --- | --- |

Total     **/22**

## Learning Points

There is a useful learning module called 'organ donation' on the RCEM learning website. Familiarise yourself with the role of the specialist nurse for organ donation (SNOD) in your hospital. Organ donation is often not addressed in cases that have not involved the ITU. Remember to call the SNOD and ask them if donation is a possibility.

## Reference

https://www.rcemlearning.co.uk/foamed/organ-donation/

## 6.5 **Difficult Referral**

### Instructions for Candidate

You are the night registrar in the ED and have a 74-year-old man in Resus with a leaking AAA. He presented complaining of loin-to-groin pain and a collapse. His BP is 90 mmHg systolic and his focused assessment with sonography for trauma (FAST) scan shows a 6 cm aneurysm with free fluid.

You have established wide-bore access and activated the major haemorrhage protocol. You have the ITU registrar with you who is preparing for transfer. Unfortunately, your hospital does not have a vascular surgeon on call tonight, and the surgical registrar is currently in theatre.

The patient walks three miles per day and suffers from hypertension only.

Please refer the patient to the surgical registrar on call at the receiving hospital.

### Mark Scheme Breakdown

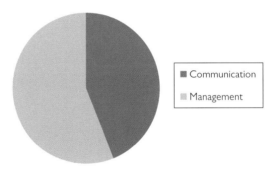

**Figure 6.5.1** Difficult referral mark scheme breakdown.

### Instructions for Actor

You are a colorectal SpR on call at the receiving hospital. You are tired and have just finished a laparotomy. The consultant vascular surgeon on call tonight is notoriously unpleasant and you do not want to wake them up.

You want the patient to have a CT scan before leaving as you are concerned that if you call the vascular consultant and the patient does not have a AAA after all, you will be in trouble. You also want the local surgical registrar to review the patient before the patient is transferred and to refer directly to the vascular consultant on call.

If the ED registrar explains the situation, you will see sense and accept the patient. If they become rude, communication will be broken down and the confrontation will escalate.

### Instructions for Examiner

Observation only.

# Equipment Required

None.

# Mark Scheme

| | |
|---|---|
| Introduces self by name and grade, and confirms who they are | |
| Explains would like to discuss a patient with a leaking AAA for urgent transfer | |
| Provides a history with salient points: patient's ID, the presentation, past medical history, and examination and FAST scan findings | |
| Describes the patient's current status: he is not intubated but is being optimised for transfer as soon as possible | |
| Explains the clinical concerns and why it is not appropriate to perform a CT scan before transfer | |
| Gives the surgical SpR the opportunity to explain their concerns and reasons | |
| Acknowledges the SpR's concerns | |
| Explains the need for prompt transfer so as not to delay emergency surgery | |
| Explains that it is not in the patient's best interest to wait for a local surgical review prior to transfer (local SpR is unavailable in theatre) | |
| Offers to speak to the vascular consultant directly | |
| Explains that the patient needs to be transferred by ambulance with an ITU escort now. Failure to do so could cause harm to the patient | |
| Maintains patient safety and well-being as the priority throughout the referral | |
| Remains professional and polite | |
| Successfully negotiates the situation and gets consent for transfer | |

Total    /**14**

# Learning Points

This case highlights the importance of using your communication and negotiation skills to advocate for the patient so that optimal care can be given. You need to demonstrate to the examiner that you are confident in your clinical assessment and in developing a management plan and that you can communicate this clearly and politely in order to ensure your referral is accepted. Acknowledge that sometimes there is a difference in opinion between colleagues regarding the best management, but this can be discussed professionally. Recognition of the human factors at play—both for you and the receiving specialist—may help the negotiation and improve the outcome, i.e. acceptance of the referral.

## 6.6 **Immunisation Refusal**

### Instructions for Candidate

An emergency nurse practitioner (ENP) has assessed George, a seven-year-old boy who presented with a rusty nail injury to his foot. The nail was in a manure heap into which the boy fell whilst climbing over a fence yesterday. George has been brought in as the wound is red and inflamed. Your colleague has washed the wound, given antibiotics, and referred to the orthopaedics team. She has asked you to speak to the family as they are refusing tetanus immunisation. George is unvaccinated and lives on a farm.

### Mark Scheme Breakdown

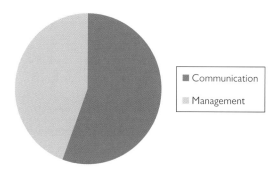

**Figure 6.6.1** Immunizations refusal mark scheme breakdown.

### Instructions for Actor

You do not want your son to have any vaccinations as you are concerned that you can catch the disease against which you are immunising from the vaccine. You have heard that some vaccines cause autism and may harm George. George had his first baby immunisations and had a temperature, rash, and febrile convulsion, and you have not given him any immunisations since. You do not know what tetanus disease is and think that people do not really catch it anymore.

### Instructions for Examiner

Observation only.

### Equipment Required

None.

# Mark Scheme

| | |
|---|---|
| Introduces self and confirms their identities and relationship | |
| Confirms a brief history of events and acknowledges the wound occurred yesterday from a dirty nail covered in manure | |
| Explains why George needs the tetanus vaccination and tetanus immunoglobulin | |
| Explains what tetanus disease is and the serious nature of the infection | |
| Elicits mum's concerns | |
| Explains that the tetanus vaccine is not a live vaccine and that George cannot catch tetanus disease from it | |
| Explains and reassures that the vaccine does not cause seizures or autism | |
| Explains what a febrile convulsion is and that it is due to the fever | |
| Reassures mum that the tetanus vaccine is not associated with a fever | |
| Explains that the incubation period is 4–14 days, and that because the wound was contaminated and treatment has been delayed until today, there is a higher risk of getting tetanus | |
| Remains non-confrontational | |
| Explores if there are any further ideas, concerns, and expectations | |
| Answers any remaining questions | |
| Negotiates and agrees on a management plan | |
| Advises mum that George will need to complete the course via the GP | |
| Provides mum with literature to read | |
| Demonstrates a good rapport with mum and George | |

Total    /**18**

# Learning Points

Success in this station requires you to know the routine immunisation schedule, as well as the management of tetanus-prone wounds. You will need to address the mother's concerns regarding vaccines, febrile convulsions, and autism. Acknowledge that you both want what is best for the child. Provide her with the correct information that she needs to make an informed decision. The manner in which this is done is crucial to arriving at a joint decision.

# References

https://www.gov.uk/government/publications/the-complete-routine-immunisation-schedule
https://assets.publishing.service.gov.uk/government/uploads/system/uploads/attachment_data/file/859519/
    Greenbook_chapter_30_Tetanus_January_2020.pdf

## 6.7 **Driving after a Seizure**

### Instructions for Candidate

You have seen a 48-year-old lady following a first fit today. You have taken a history and examined her and will make a referral to the first fit clinic. Please tell the patient that she needs to inform the DVLA and must stop driving immediately.

### Mark Scheme Breakdown

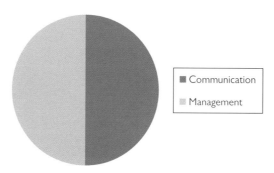

**Figure 6.7.1** Driving advice after a seizure mark scheme breakdown.

### Instructions for Actor

You are a drug rep from Wales, and you drive many miles per week as part of your job. Today you were visiting the hospital for work when you had a fit in the car park. You had been out partying last night and did not have very much sleep.

When the doctor informs you that you are no longer able to drive, you become very upset and irrational. You do not believe you will have another fit as it was probably because of alcohol excess and sleep deprivation and you will stop partying. You refuse to inform the DVLA or stop driving.

When the doctor informs you that if you drive, you will not be insured and that you would be criminally liable in an accident, you sit down and listen and apologise. You are very worried how you will pay the bills now.

If the doctor does not explain the situation adequately and does not establish a good rapport, you storm out.

### Instructions for Examiner

Observation only.

### Equipment Required

None.

# Mark Scheme

| | |
|---|---|
| Clarifies the patient's understanding of the diagnosis and management so far | |
| Explains the risk of having a further seizure whilst driving | |
| Sensitively explains that she needs to stop driving immediately and must inform the DVLA | |
| Acknowledges her upset and shows empathy | |
| Confirms the patient's occupation | |
| Explains that driving after a seizure against medical advice will invalidate her insurance and she may be criminally liable if she has an accident | |
| Explains that she will not be able to drive for six months unless told otherwise by the neurologist following review in the first fit clinic | |
| Assures the patient that these rules are to ensure her safety and the safety of others on the road | |
| Explains that this discussion will be documented in the notes and relayed to her GP | |
| Encourages the patient to adhere to the advice and inform the DVLA herself | |
| Sensitively explains that failure to comply would result in informing the DVLA on the patient's behalf | |
| Provides seizure safety advice regarding alcohol, swimming, or bathing alone, using machinery, working at heights, etc. | |
| Provides a patient information leaflet and reiterates the follow-up plan | |
| Elicits any other concerns and invites further questions | |
| Summarises and ends the consultation | |
| Establishes good rapport and shows empathy and sensitivity | |

Total    /**16**

# Learning Points

The link from the DVLA (see References below) provides guidance on medical conditions and the DVLA advice/driving restrictions. Note the difference for category 1 and 2 drivers.

# Reference

https://assets.publishing.service.gov.uk/government/uploads/system/uploads/attachment_data/file/834504/assessing-fitness-to-drive-a-guide-for-medical-professionals.pdf

## 6.8 **Conflict with a Colleague**

### Instructions for Candidate

An ST3 trainee who is new to the department comes to you with some images they have taken during a FAST scan. They are currently trying to complete their ultrasound portfolio for sign-off. The patient is a 79-year-old man presenting with back and groin pain. Please review the images with them and answer their questions.

### Mark Scheme Breakdown

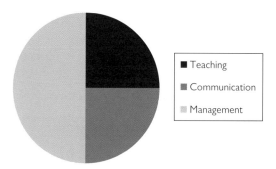

**Figure 6.8.1** Conflict with colleague mark scheme breakdown.

### Instructions for Actor

You are a keen Emergency Medicine ST3. You have just finished your ITU training and feel like you are extremely competent and experienced. You completed your USS training level 1 course and you are trying to collect cases for your portfolio to be signed off.

You really want the registrar to sign you off for AAA scanning now. You feel affronted when the registrar points out your error, and you keep asking to have a case signed off, even though you mis-interpreted the scan.

### Instructions for Examiner

Observation only.

### Equipment Required

Ultrasound image (Fig. 6.8.2).

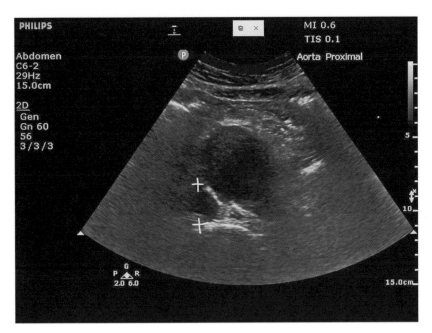

**Figure 6.8.2** Ultrasound image case 6.8.

## Mark Scheme

| | |
|---|---|
| Introduces self to the doctor and confirms their name and grade | |
| Asks if the ST3 needs help | |
| Listens to the history and looks at the scan images provided | |
| Notices that the ST3 has misinterpreted the scan and missed the large aneurysm in the corner of the image | |
| Asks where the patient is, checks he is safe, and requests a senior colleague to review him immediately | |
| Provides teaching on the scan and indicates where the aorta is on the image | |
| Constructively explains that the structure measured by the ST3 is, in fact, the inferior vena cava | |
| Acknowledges the desire for the portfolio to be signed off but states that, in this case, that would not be appropriate | |
| Recommends further supervised scanning and learning | |
| Arranges a time to help with this and signposts to colleagues who can help with supervised scanning as well | |
| Asks if there are any final questions | |

Total    /**11**

## Learning Points

You are expected to be competent at performing point-of-care ultrasound. If you are not using it frequently in your clinical practice, familiarise yourself before the exam. We recommend you complete the learning modules on ultrasound in emergency medicine on the RCEM learning website.

Do not be pressured into signing off an assessment if, as in this case, the trainee is not yet competent at performing the skill. Recognise it as an opportunity for ongoing development. Most importantly, however, you must ensure patient safety.

## Reference

https://www.rcemlearning.co.uk/reference/ultrasound-in-emergency-medicine-level-1-instruction

## 6.9 **Angry Relative**

### Instructions for Candidate

Sister has asked you to talk to Mrs Batten as she is very angry. Her son had an X-ray taken three hours ago and the doctor has not come back to talk to her since. The SHO who attended the patient and requested the X-ray has gone home and did not hand the patient over. Please go and talk to Mrs Batten and resolve the situation.

### Mark Scheme Breakdown

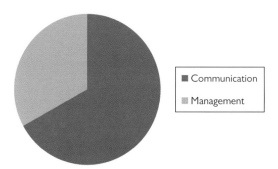

**Figure 6.9.1** Angry relative mark scheme breakdown.

### Instructions for Actor

You are incredibly angry. You brought your seven-year-old son in with a painful hip four hours ago. Your son has not had any further pain relief since being given paracetamol at triage. He was seen by an SHO who sent him for an X-ray and he has not been back to see you since. You have been sitting here patiently for three hours and now your son is in more pain. You want to know what is going on.

If the doctor acknowledges a mistake has been made, as the SHO went home and forgot to hand the patient over, and shows empathy and offers analgesia and appropriate management, you calm down. If they do not establish a good rapport and apologise, you remain very angry and will make a formal complaint.

### Instructions for Examiner

Observation only.

### Equipment Required

X-ray pelvis (Fig. 6.9.2).

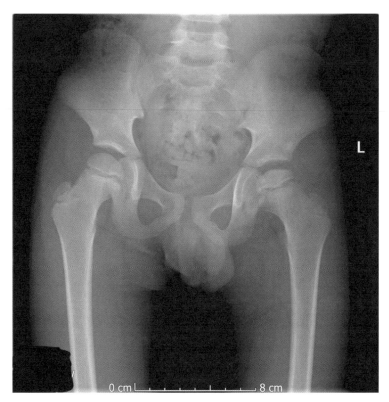

**Figure 6.9.2** X-ray pelvis case 6.9.

## Mark Scheme

| | |
|---|---|
| Introduces self, confirms the names of the child and mother | |
| Allows the mother to explain her concerns uninterrupted | |
| Apologises for the long wait and acknowledges that an error has been made | |
| Explains that the patient was not handed over and that it is understandable that she is upset | |
| Demonstrates empathy | |
| Reassures mum that her complaint is taken very seriously | |
| Reassures mum that the SHO will be spoken to | |
| Reassures mum that the importance of handover will be reiterated to the whole team | |

| | |
|---|---|
| Offers analgesia | |
| Offers to help and treat her son now | |
| Correctly interprets the X-ray which shows Perthes' disease | |
| Explains the diagnosis to mum | |
| Explains the management plan | |
| Asks if she has any questions or further concerns | |
| If mum is still unhappy, provides information for formal complaint via Patient Advice and Liaison Service (PALS) | |
| Establishes a good rapport and diffuses the situation successfully | |

Total    /**16**

## Learning Points

Acknowledge that a mistake has been made and that the mother is understandably angry and upset. Not only have they been missed and forgotten about, but the child is in pain, and they have just received news of a new diagnosis. Apologise, offer analgesia, and allow plenty of time for explanations and empathy.

Be familiar with X-ray interpretation for Perthes' disease and other differentials, e.g. slipped upper femoral epiphysis (SUFE). Be able to explain these diagnoses and the initial management and follow-up to a parent. A reminder of common causes of childhood limp by age is included in Table 6.9.1 for reference.

**Table 6.9.1** Causes of a limp in children

| All ages | Toddlers (age 1–3) | Age 4–10 | Adolescents (age 11–16) |
|---|---|---|---|
| Septic arthritis | Developmental | Transient synovitis | Slipped upper femoral |
| Osteomyelitis | dysplasia of the hip | (most common | epiphysis |
| Trauma (fractures, soft | Toddler's fractures | age 3–5) | Osteochondritis |
| tissue injuries, foreign | (non-displaced spiral | Perthes' disease | Gonococcal septic arthritis |
| bodies) | fracture of lower third | Leukaemia | (see Section 5.11) |
| Neoplasm (the distal | of tibia) | | Physeal injuries |
| femoral epiphyseal | Transient synovitis | | Ewing's sarcoma |
| plate is the fastest- | (most common | | |
| growing area of bone | age 3–5) | | |
| and at high risk of | | | |
| neoplasm) | | | |
| Sickle cell crisis | | | |
| Neuromuscular | | | |
| (e.g. cerebral palsy, | | | |
| Duchenne muscular | | | |
| dystrophy) | | | |
| Juvenile arthritis | | | |
| Henoch–Schönlein | | | |
| purpura | | | |
| Referred pain (e.g. from | | | |
| the abdomen) | | | |
| Non-accidental injury | | | |

# Reference

Banerjee A, Oliver C (2017) *Revision Notes for the FRCEM Intermediate SAQ Paper*, 2nd edition. Oxford University Press: Oxford.

## 6.10 **New Diagnosis**

### Instructions for Candidate

An eight-year-old boy presented with his mother, having collapsed at school. He came in drowsy and dehydrated, with abdominal pain and vomiting. He was found to have diabetic ketoacidosis (DKA), and a new diagnosis of type 1 diabetes was confirmed and is being treated. The mother is currently unaware of the diagnosis of diabetes, although she knows he came in with a high blood sugar. Please explain the diagnosis and answer any questions.

### Mark Scheme Breakdown

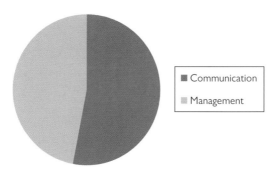

**Figure 6.10.1** New diagnosis mark scheme breakdown.

### Instructions for Actor

Your son was brought in very unwell after he collapsed at school. You have been told he has been treated for a high blood sugar and dehydration. You are not aware that this means he is diabetic. You have no understanding of what diabetes is, although you did have a grandmother with diabetes, but she just had to stop eating sugary foods. In retrospect, you had noticed that he was drinking and passing urine all the time, and now you feel guilty you did not notice he was ill.

You are very nervous about having to administer insulin and do not think you will be able to do this. When it is explained that your son is being admitted and before discharge, you will have lots of training and written advice on what to do and access to the specialist nurse, you feel reassured.

### Instructions for Examiner

Observation only.

### Equipment Required

None.

## Mark Scheme

| | |
|---|---|
| Introduces self to the patient and mum | |
| Confirms child's name and mother's name and their relationship | |
| Clarifies what they know so far | |
| Clarifies key aspects of the history | |
| Sensitively explains that the diagnosis is type 1 diabetes | |
| Asks what they know about the condition | |
| Explains what diabetes is | |
| Explains the treatment that has been given so far | |
| Acknowledges that this is a life-altering diagnosis and offers support | |
| Explains what will happen next: | |
| • Admission to the paediatric ward | |
| • Ongoing treatment for DKA and diabetes | |
| Explores their ideas, concerns, and expectations | |
| Answers questions appropriately | |
| Provides further sources of information, e.g. leaflets, support groups, or recommended websites | |
| Explains that mum and child will be taught how to manage the condition, including how to give insulin | |
| Reassures mum that there will be regular follow-up with the specialist nurse and follow-up in clinic | |
| Checks understanding of the discussion | |
| Invites final questions | |
| Establishes good rapport with mum and child | |

Total    /**19**

## Learning Points

Some candidates struggle with communication stations if it is not a natural skill. However, it really is possible to score well with practice. It is common in the FRCEM OSCE that you will have to explain a diagnosis and management plan to the patient. Practise doing this in exam style at work. Remember to avoid using medical jargon, take cues from the patient, and always address their ideas, concerns, and expectations. A summary at the end is helpful. Allow the patient to ask questions. Do not be put off if you are not particularly familiar with a condition—just explain in layman's terms.

## 6.11 **Assessing Capacity**

### Instructions for Candidate

You are the night registrar and have been asked by the SHO for some help to manage a patient that they feel does not have capacity and is trying to leave. They have severe cellulitis of their lower leg and require intravenous antibiotics.

The patient is a 78-year-old lifelong farmer. He lives by himself and is very keen to get back as he needs to feed the animals and put them away for the night. He was sent in by his sister who was concerned that he was acting strangely. His sister has called to say she will get a neighbour to help with the animals and then will come to the hospital.

Please speak to the patient, assess his capacity, and formulate a management plan.

### Mark Scheme Breakdown

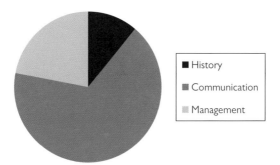

**Figure 6.11.1** Assessing capacity mark scheme breakdown.

### Instructions for Actor

You have been a farmer all your life and you never see a doctor. You are angry that your sister has sent you in and do not feel there is anything wrong with you. You do not really know where you are and think you may be in prison. When it is explained to you that you are in hospital, you are not happy and try to leave. You do not like doctors or ill people.

You did not know you had cellulitis, although your leg is hurting. When the diagnosis and risks are explained to you, you do not really understand and cannot remember what was just explained to you. You are confused about the day and year and are having visual hallucinations. You keep picking at dirty marks on your clothes and thinking that they are buttons that need to be done up.

You calm down a little when it is explained to you that the animals are being taken care of by your neighbour. You trust him as he is also a farmer.

# Instructions for Examiner

Observation only.

# Equipment Required

None.

# Mark Scheme

| | |
|---|---|
| Introduces self to the patient and confirms his identity | |
| Asks if he is comfortable and offers analgesia | |
| Asks the patient if he knows why he is here | |
| Checks the patient is orientated in time, place, and person | |
| Reassures the patient that he is not in prison and is in hospital | |
| Explains the diagnosis and the treatment | |
| Explains the risks of not being treated | |
| Explores why he does not want to stay and have treatment | |
| Tries to alleviate some of the patient's concerns regarding his animals | |
| Assesses whether the patient can balance the risks and benefits | |
| Assesses if the patient can understand, retain, and weigh the diagnosis and the risks, and whether he can communicate his decision | |
| Explains that he is not well and that he is being admitted for treatment | |
| Reassures the patient that the treatment will help him to feel better | |
| Reassures the patient that he will be better able to look after his animals once the cellulitis is improving | |
| Reassures the patient that his sister is coming in to see him and offers the opportunity to talk again when she arrives | |
| Answers any questions | |
| Establishes a rapport and explains matters clearly to the patient | |
| Notes that a full Mini-Mental State Examination (MMSE) needs to be performed | |
| Thanks the patient and ensures he is comfortable | |

Total    /**19**

## Learning Points

The Mental Capacity Act (2005) and how it is used to assess capacity is discussed in Section 8.1. Success in this station is not simply about assessing capacity. You must demonstrate to the examiner that you have a patient-centred approach. Ensure the patient is comfortable. Use your communication skills to provide explanations in a way that he will understand. Determine what the patient's main concerns are. Attempt to reassure and alleviate any concerns (no matter how trivial they may seem) that may interfere with his decision-making. Even if a patient is deemed to lack capacity, your communication skills can help reduce distress and improve the patient experience during a difficult situation.

# Chapter 7 **Resuscitation Scenarios**

# The Resuscitation Station

There are two double stations in the FRCEM OSCE and these tend to be an ALS-based resuscitation scenario such as a cardiac arrest and a trauma case. They can be adult or paediatric. It is common for these to have a further focus such as breaking bad news, debriefing the team, or dealing with a difficult team or family member. They will sometimes incorporate a teaching element such as talking someone through how to insert a chest drain or an IO line during the scenario.

The simulations are low-tech, and the helpers are very efficient and generally competent, although be wary of a scenario where the 'extra something' is an incompetent team member.

It is important to review the pie chart of how the marks are divided, so that you do not get carried away in the scenario and miss vital points.

The following scenarios are best practised as a group in a simulation suite if you have access to one, which is how we (the authors) prepared.

# 7.1 **Advanced Life Support 1**

This is a double station.

## Instructions for Candidate

A 52-year-old gentleman has just been found collapsed in the car park. He had been discharged from the ED 20 minutes earlier by an advanced care practitioner (ACP), after presenting earlier that day with chest pain. Please resuscitate the patient and then hot debrief the team, including the ACP. You have two ED nurses, an ED registrar, and the same ACP to assist you.

## Mark Scheme Breakdown

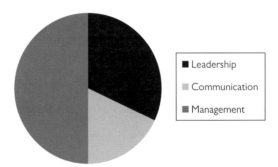

**Figure 7.1.1** Advanced life support 1 mark scheme breakdown.

## Instructions for Actor

*ED Nurses 1 and 2*

You are competent and can follow clear instructions. If the candidate does not suggest rotating for CPR, you tire and your compressions become ineffective. You are able to use the defibrillator safely.

*ED Registrar*

You are confident to manage the airway and are keen to intubate if required. If asked to undertake intubation, you initially have an (unrecognised) oesophageal intubation. If this is recognised by the candidate, you succeed on your next attempt at intubation.

*ACP*

You are upset and tearful that you had discharged the patient home. You try to help the resuscitation efforts, but you keep dropping things and keep speaking over the candidate. If asked for further information, you state that he had presented with chest pain after heavy lifting and you had thought it was musculoskeletal pain. The ECG was unremarkable. No blood tests were taken.

## Instructions for Examiner

The patient is in cardiac arrest, with an initial rhythm of ventricular fibrillation (VF). He remains in VF until after the third shock/adrenaline and amiodarone have been administered, at which point there is return of spontaneous circulation (ROSC). If the candidate fails to recognise the initial oesophageal intubation or fails to secure the airway, then the patient will go into asystole and resuscitation efforts will be futile.

Prompt the candidate at ten minutes (if resuscitation is not concluded) to debrief the team and feed back to the ACP. Ask the candidate for further management of the missed diagnosis outside of the Resus room.

## Equipment Required

An equipped SIM suite.

## Mark Scheme

| | |
|---|---|
| Introduces self to the team and takes role as the team leader | |
| Establishes the patient is in cardiac arrest, initiates CPR, and attaches the defibrillator | |
| **Correctly identifies the rhythm as VF and safely administers the shock to the patient** | |
| **Correctly works through the four Hs and four Ts** | |
| Swaps team members for CPR and/or identifies ineffective CPR | |
| Establishes/requests a secure airway with $ETCO_2$ monitoring | |
| Recognises and corrects the oesophageal intubation | |
| **Gives correct drugs and doses at the correct time** | |
| Uses the team effectively | |
| Manages the upset ACP during arrest and advises standing back | |
| Recognises ROSC and instigates post-resuscitation care | |
| Requests cardiology and intensive care input | |
| **Facilitates a constructive debrief** | |
| Is non-judgemental and provides feedback to the team and ACP | |
| Further management of the case when asked by examiner: | |
| Will raise an incident form | |
| Should state that this will be investigated as a serious incident | |
| Duty of candour to patient and family | |

| | |
|---|---|
| Information gathering: secures and copies the notes from the earlier encounter, asks the ACP to write a statement of what happened, identifies other staff members involved, and gets their version of events | |
| Immediate management of the ACP: are they safe to continue working? When are their next duties? Do other patients need to be reviewed? | |
| Ongoing management of the ACP: inform the ACP's supervisor—determine whether this was an isolated case or if there are further concerns | |
| Consideration of further education for the ACP and the wider team | |
| Checks that departmental guidelines are appropriate and accessible | |
| **Displays effective team leadership skills** | |

*NB Up to 2 marks available for actions in bold.*

Total    **/28**

# Learning Points

This is a seemingly straightforward ALS scenario where you are expected to manage a cardiac arrest as per ALS guidelines, and then manage the post-ROSC scenario. However, a significant portion of the marks is given for handling the ACP during the scenario and the management of this once the clinical scenario is finished. Valuable marks would be lost, even if the ALS scenario was managed effectively, if you allowed yourself to become distracted by the ACP and did not know how to deal with a serious incident. Again, look at the pie chart carefully and maintain awareness of the actors in the room and the distractions they throw at you.

# References

https://www.rcem.ac.uk/docs/Safety/82d.%20Safe-Leadership.pdf
https://www.resus.org.uk/resuscitation-guidelines/adult-advanced-life-support/
https://www.rcem.ac.uk/RCEM/Exams_Training/Emergency_Care_ACP/RCEM/Exams_Training/
   Emergency_Care_ACP/Emergency_Care_ACP.aspx

## 7.2  **Advanced Life Support 2**

This is a double station.

## Instructions for Candidate

A 54-year-old lady has been brought into Resus after an overdose of her own medication. Three empty packets of propranolol were brought in by the paramedics. She has a reduced conscious level and is hypotensive and bradycardic.

## Mark Scheme Breakdown

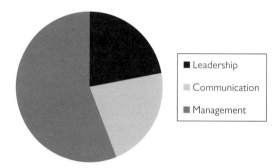

**Figure 7.2.1**  Adult life support 2 mark scheme breakdown.

## Instructions for Actor

*ITU Registrar*

You arrive once the patient has ROSC. The unit is full and you are overwhelmed with referrals. In addition, the ITU consultant on call today is a notorious bully. As a result, you do not want to accept the patient and are obstructive and rude to the candidate.

## Instructions for Examiner

Please provide the clinical findings as the candidate assesses the patient:

A: partially obstructed. Corrects with airway manoeuvres/adjuncts.

B: RR 16; SaO₂ 93% on air, 100% on high flow.

C: HR 34, radial pulse not palpable, BP 64/30. ECG if requested—wide QRS.

D: GCS E2V3M5. Pupils equal, 5 mm. Blood glucose 16.2 mmol/l.

E: temperature 36.8°C.

After the A–E assessment or two minutes, the patient goes into cardiac arrest, with an initial rhythm of pulseless electrical activity (PEA) (slow). Achieve ROSC after two cycles of PEA. Prompt the candidate to refer to the ITU registrar if not already done so (ten minutes in).

## Equipment Required

An equipped SIM suite.
An arterial blood gas (Table 7.2.1).

**Table 7.2.1** Arterial blood gas results.

| pH | 7.01 |
|---|---|
| $pCO_2$ | 6.9 kPa |
| $pO_2$ | 14.5 kPa |
| ctHb | 141 g/l |
| $cK^+$ | 4.1 mmol/l |
| $cNa^+$ | 147 mmol/l |
| $cCa^{2+}$ | 1.19 mmol/l |
| $cCl^-$ | 103 mmol/l |
| cGlu | 7.0 mmol/l |
| cLac | 9.8 mmol/l |
| $cHCO_3^-$ | 16.8 mmol/l |
| cCr | 105 mmol/l |

## Mark Scheme

| | |
|---|---|
| Introduces self to team and takes role as team leader | |
| Asks for further help | |
| Performs A–E assessment: | |
| • A: airway manoeuvres and/or adjuncts | |
| • B: high-flow $O_2$ | |

| | |
|---|---|
| • C: IV access secured, ECG or cardiac monitoring. Appropriate drug(s), bradycardia management, and fluids given<br>Acceptable drugs/treatment: atropine, sodium bicarbonate 8.4%, dobutamine, isoprenaline, glucagon or insulin/dextrose, or transthoracic pacing | |
| • D: assesses GCS and blood glucose | |
| • E: exposure | |
| Recognises and confirms patient is in cardiac arrest | |
| **Correctly identifies rhythm as PEA and follows non-shockable side of ALS algorithm** | |
| **Correctly works through the four Hs and four Ts (toxins)** | |
| **Considers appropriate management of propranolol overdose: 8.4% sodium bicarbonate, intralipid, high-dose insulin, awareness that prolonged resuscitation may be appropriate** | |
| Establishes/requests secure airway | |
| Recognises ROSC and initiates post-resuscitation care | |
| Requests intensive care input | |
| Uses the team effectively | |
| Referral: | |
| • Introduces self and checks identity of ITU SpR | |
| • States the intention to refer the patient | |
| • Gives a clear, structured handover | |
| Remains calm and professional despite provocation | |
| Calmly negotiates the need for this patient to go to ITU | |
| Suggests escalation to the ED consultant and/or ITU consultant if referral still refused | |
| Demonstrates an understanding of ITU SpR's situation and tries to alleviate issues where possible | |
| **Displays effective team leadership skills** | |

*NB Up to 2 marks available for actions in bold.*

Total    /**27**

## Learning Points

Toxicology features quite commonly in the OSCE in various formats. Read around the management of drugs of overdose on TOXBASE® and be familiar with antidotes and management. We suggest being familiar with tricyclic antidepressants, selective serotonin reuptake inhibitors (SSRIs), paracetamol, ethylene glycol, beta-blockers, calcium channel blockers, and opiates as a bare minimum.

## References

https://www.toxbase.org/
https://em3.org.uk/foamed/23/3/2016/beta-blocker-od

## 7.3 **Newborn Life Support**

This is a double station.

## Instructions for Candidate

A term infant has just been born in the ED. Please assess and resuscitate the infant as required. You have a competent ED nurse with you. Please explain the news to the infant's father when he arrives.

## Mark Scheme Breakdown

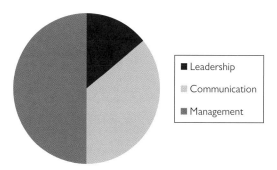

**Figure 7.3.1** Newborn life support mark scheme breakdown.

## Instructions for Actor

*ED Nurse*

You know where equipment is kept and will follow any instructions given, but show no initiative.

*Father of Child*

It is your first child and you have just relocated to the area and speak minimal English. You are very frightened and upset and concerned about your baby. You decline a translator, but if the candidate speaks too quickly or uses medical jargon, then you get annoyed and agitated.

## Instructions for Examiner

The child is blue and floppy, making no respiratory effort, and has a HR of 50 bpm. The mother is being looked after by another doctor.

The chest does not rise until the candidate has used an airway adjunct and a two-person technique for the five inflation breaths. The HR remains at 50 bpm until after 30 seconds of chest compressions have been completed, at which point the baby starts to cry and the HR rises to >100 bpm.

Ask the candidate to explain what has happened to the infant's father.

# Equipment Required

Flat surface (no Resuscitaire® available).
Towels, hat.
Stop clock.
Airway kit: appropriate size masks, bag–valve–mask (BVM), oropharyngeal airway, suction.
Baby mannequin.

# Mark Scheme

| | |
|---|---|
| Appropriate introduction to the nurse and team | |
| Calls for help: requests neonatal resuscitation team | |
| Checks that the mother is safe and being cared for by colleagues | |
| Dries the baby and then discards the wet towel | |
| Starts the clock | |
| Wraps the baby in a dry towel and places a hat on the baby's head | |
| Assesses colour and tone | |
| Assess breathing and HR | |
| Opens the airway: neutral position | |
| **Gives five inflation breaths with BVM and continually assesses if chest rising** | |
| Requests SpO$_2$ monitoring (pre-ductal) and cardiac monitoring | |
| **Notes there is no chest rise or increase in HR and repositions, uses adjuncts or a two-person technique until sees chest rise** | |
| Once the chest is rising, notes the HR is still slow (<60 bpm) and gives 30 seconds' ventilation breaths | |
| Reassess the HR: notes the HR is still slow and starts CPR at ratio of 3:1 for 30 seconds | |
| Reassesses and notes the improved HR and condition of infant | |
| Hands over to the neonatal team | |
| **Demonstrates a structured approach as per newborn life support (NLS) algorithm** | |
| Introduces self to the father and explains role | |
| Checks understanding/what they know so far | |

| | |
|---|---|
| Offers a translator or alternative, adjusts speech, and avoids jargon | |
| **Explains the resuscitation of the infant and the need for further observation** | |
| **Allows the opportunity for questions and answers appropriately** | |
| Closes the conversation appropriately | |

*NB Up to 2 marks available for actions in bold.*

Total   **/28**

# Learning Points

This station gives you the opportunity to demonstrate your knowledge of the NLS algorithm (Fig. 7.3.2), as well as your communication skills under stressful circumstances.

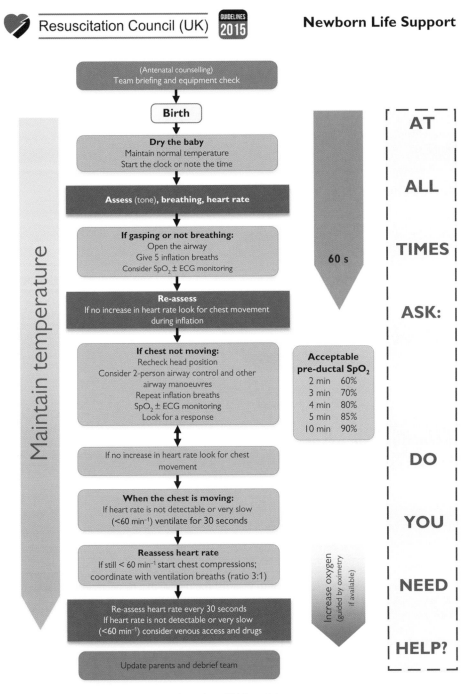

**Figure 7.3.2** Newborn life support algorithm, 2015 guidelines.

Reproduced with the kind permission of the Resuscitation Council (UK).

## 7.4 **Adult Trauma 1**

This is a double station.

### Instructions for Candidate

A 61-year-old farmer has just been brought in after being trampled on by a cow. He has self-presented through Minors and the triage nurse has asked you to see him as she is concerned as he is pale and breathless.

### Mark Scheme Breakdown

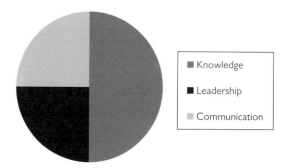

**Figure 7.4.1** Adult trauma mark scheme breakdown.

### Instructions for Actor

*ED Nurses 1 and 2*

You are competent and can follow clear instructions.

*ED ST3*

You are keen to get involved and want to do any procedures. You have done an ATLS course and inserted a chest drain once before under direct supervision.

*Surgical SpR*

You do not want to take this man straight to theatre. You believe that he needs further imaging first and that either conservative management or interventional radiology is more appropriate.

### Instructions for Examiner

When requested, the following parameters are available:

- A: patent.
- B: RR 30; SaO$_2$ 90% on air, 94% on high flow. Unequal chest movement and an obvious deformity to the chest wall. Bruised and tender to palpation. There is reduced air entry on the left. Dull to percussion.

- C: HR 104, BP 102/68. Looks pale. Abdomen is soft, but tender in epigastrium and left upper quadrant (LUQ). Pelvis is apparently normal and there are no long bone injuries. If a FAST scan is undertaken, there is a rim of free fluid in the LUQ view.
- D: GCS E4V5M6. Pupils equal, 3 mm. Blood glucose 6.1 mmol/l.
- E: temperature 36.8°C. No other obvious injuries.

If the candidate wishes to place an intercostal drain, ask them to teach the CT3 how to do it. The patient stabilises after the chest drain has been inserted and two units of blood have been transfused.

## Equipment Required

An equipped SIM suite.
CXR (Fig. 7.4.2).

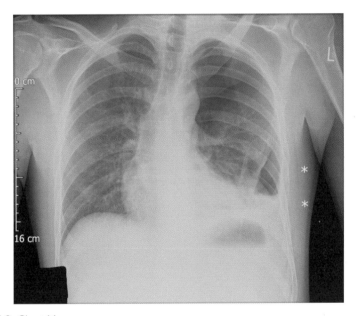

**Figure 7.4.2** Chest X-ray.

## Mark Scheme

| | |
|---|---|
| Introduces self and takes role as the team leader | |
| Ensures the patient is moved into Resus and activates the hospital trauma team | |
| Offers analgesia to the patient | |
| Briefs the team and allocates roles | |
| Completes the primary survey | |
| **Obtains an AMPLE history** | |

| | |
|---|---|
| Requests high-flow $O_2$ | |
| Recognises chest injury | |
| Requests a primary survey CXR and correctly interprets it (pneumohaemothorax and multiple rib fractures) | |
| Requests a chest drain | |
| Talks the ST3 through how to insert the chest drain: | |
| • Asks about previous experience | |
| • Uses a safety checklist, confirms with the CXR and the examination to ensure the correct side is used | |
| • Adequate analgesia: considers sedation | |
| • Explains the procedure to the patient and obtains verbal consent | |
| • Prepares the equipment | |
| • Local anaesthetic (if conscious) | |
| • Explains the landmarks / safe triangle | |
| • Makes incision to avoid neurovascular bundle | |
| • Uses blunt dissection and a finger sweep | |
| • Sites the chest drain and connects to the underwater seal | |
| • Confirms the drain is swinging and draining | |
| • Sutures the chest drain in place | |
| • States the need to check the post-procedure CXR | |
| • Disposes of sharps safely | |
| Administers tranexamic acid | |
| Appropriate resuscitation with blood products | |
| **Has a discussion with the team about further management and decides a reasonable management plan** <br> **(There is no 'correct' plan, so points awarded on decision-making, rationale, and quality of discussion with team/surgical SpR)** | |
| Gives constructive debrief and thanks team | |
| Displays effective team leadership skills | |

*NB Up to 2 marks available for actions in bold.*

Total    /**31**

## Learning Points

Be familiar with all practical procedures related to trauma such as insertion of chest drain, obtaining IO access, application of splints, and haemorrhage control.

This station initially seems to be a straightforward ATLS scenario, but the candidate will soon be expected to recognise there are other elements—in this case, teaching, conflict resolution, communication skills, and complex decision-making. Be prepared to defend and negotiate the plan, where appropriate, to provide optimal care for the patient. Be polite and professional.

## 7.5  **Advanced Paediatric Life Support**

This is a double station.

## Instructions for Candidate

A 13-month old who is seizing has been phoned through to the department. The paramedics have noticed a bruise near the child's ear and are concerned about a possible head injury. You have two minutes to prepare for the child's arrival.

## Mark Scheme Breakdown

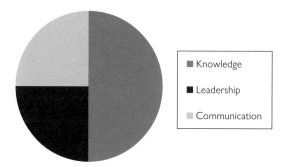

■ Knowledge

■ Leadership

▨ Communication

**Figure 7.5.1**  Advanced paediatric life support mark scheme breakdown.

## Instructions for Actor

*Paramedic*

You have brought in a child who has been fitting for 15 minutes. You have been unable to gain IV access but have administered one dose of rectal diazepam.

*Team*

You are competent and can follow clear instructions.

*Mum and Partner (not the Child's Father)*

You arrive on the examiner's nod. You are difficult to engage with and do not make eye contact. You do not know how the bruise occurred. If the issue of non-accidental injury is raised, you become angry and defensive.

## Instructions for Examiner

When requested, the following parameters are available:

• A: secretions which clear with suctioning.

- B: RR 38; $SaO_2$ 92% on air, 99% on high-flow $O_2$.
- C: HR 160, CRT <2 seconds. Unable to obtain IV access on two attempts. Candidates should indicate they will use IO.
- D: still fitting. GCS E1V1M1. Pupils equal, 3 mm. Blood glucose 6.1 mmol/l.
- E: temperature 38.1°C. Bruise behind the right ear is noted. Fingertip bruises around nappy line.

After lorazepam is given, the seizure terminates, but the child stops breathing.

## Equipment Required

An equipped SIM suite.

## Mark Scheme

| | |
|---|---|
| Introduces self and takes role as the team leader | |
| Prepares to receive the child: puts out a paediatric emergency call and allocates roles | |
| WETFLAG completed appropriately. Mentions drug calculations/seizure algorithm | |
| • Weight 10 kg (allow reasonable estimate) | |
| • Energy 40 J | |
| • Tube 4/4.5 | |
| • Fluid 200 ml or 100 ml (trauma) | |
| • Lorazepam 1 mg | |
| • Adrenaline 1 ml of 1 in 10,000 | |
| • Glucose 20 ml of 10% dextrose | |
| A–E assessment undertaken: | |
| • A: applies suction and $O_2$ | |
| • B: examines the chest | |
| • C: obtains IO access and gives lorazepam | |
| • D: checks GCS, pupils, and blood sugar | |
| • E: notes fever; considers IV antibiotics. Exposes the child; looks for, and notes, bruising | |
| Reassesses the patient once the seizure has terminated | |
| **Confirms arrest: initiates five rescue breaths** | |
| **Identifies PEA and non-shockable algorithm followed** | |
| Secures the airway with an ETT | |
| Considers the four Hs and four Ts | |

| | |
|---|---|
| Identifies ROSC and starts post-resuscitation care | |
| Requests further imaging | |
| On arrival of the child's mother and mother's partner: | |
| • Introduces self to parents and checks their identity and understanding so far | |
| • Allows them to see the child, explains seizure management, then suggests going somewhere quieter to discuss events | |
| In private (ask if paediatric consultant available too): | |
| • Explains the course of events, explains the diagnosis of seizure and that concerned it could be related to an infection | |
| • Explains you are also concerned the seizure may be related to a head injury as bruises were found. Asks if they were aware of any injuries | |
| • Explains what will happen now (seizure management, CT, discussion with specialist team, discussion with safeguarding team) | |
| • Allows parents to ask questions, answers appropriately | |
| Gives constructive debrief and thanks team | |
| Displays effective team leadership skills | |

NB Up to 2 marks available for actions in bold.

Total    /**30**

# Learning Points

Please refer to the latest APLS manual for the status epilepticus guideline. Be aware of the time intervals between drugs.

At onset: manage the airway and provide $O_2$. Gain IV access, measure blood sugar and send some blood investigations, and call for senior help.

If the seizure is ongoing after five minutes, give 0.1 mg/kg IV/IO lorazepam. If IV/IO access is delayed or not possible, initially give 0.5 mg/kg of buccal midazolam or rectal diazepam.

If seizing after a further ten minutes, give a further dose of IV lorazepam 0.1 mg/kg. Do not exceed two doses of any type of benzodiazepine—this should include any prehospital doses.

If seizing after a further ten minutes, give IV phenytoin 20 mg/kg over 20 minutes.

If the patient is already taking phenytoin, consider phenobarbital 20 mg/kg IV over 20 minutes or levetiracetam or sodium valproate.

Whilst preparing phenytoin, consider giving PR paraldehyde 0.4 ml/kg, mixed with an equal volume of olive oil, to give a total of 0.8 ml/kg. Inform ITU and paediatrics of the situation.

If seizing after a further 20 minutes, proceed to RSI. APLS recommends the use of IV thiopental 4 mg/kg. In practice, propofol is frequently used.

As well as following the status epilepticus guideline, it is important to look for a cause and treat anything that is potentially reversible. Always consider hypoglycaemia, meningitis, intracranial disease, NAI, and toxicological causes. You, as a senior decision-maker, will be expected to determine if a CT head is appropriate.

# References

https://www.resus.org.uk/resuscitation-guidelines/paediatric-advanced-life-support
https://oxfordmedicine.com/view/10.1093/med/9780198784197.001.0001/med-9780198784197-chapter-15# med-9780198784197-chapter-15-div1-473

## 7.6 **Paediatric Trauma**

This is a double station.

### Instructions for Candidate

You receive the following pre-alert: a nine-year-old boy has been hit by a car whilst riding on a skateboard. He is crying and agitated, and has an open tibia/fibula fracture. You have two minutes to prepare for the child's arrival.

### Mark Scheme Breakdown

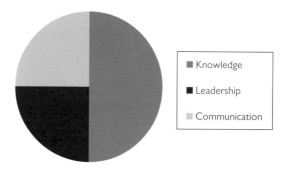

■ Knowledge

■ Leadership

▦ Communication

**Figure 7.6.1** Paediatric trauma mark scheme breakdown.

### Instructions for Actor

*Paramedic Handover*

The child skated out in front of a car travelling at approximately 30 mph. He was not wearing a helmet. Open fracture to right lower leg and has been very agitated/crying. You were unable to gain IV access. Mum is on her way in by car.

*Team*

Competent and can follow clear instructions.

*Mum*

You arrive on the examiner's nod. You are accepting of the information given but ask if your child will make a full recovery.

### Instructions for Examiner

When requested, the following parameters are available:

• A: crying.

- B: RR 28, SaO$_2$ 98% on air. Chest examination is unremarkable.
- C: HR 110, CRT <2 seconds, BP 100/65. Abdomen is soft; pelvis seems stable; small amount of bleeding from leg wound.
- D: GCS E4V3M6. Pupils equal, 3 mm. Blood glucose 6.1 mmol/l.
- E: temperature 37.1°C. Bruising to side of head and face.

If not specified, ask the candidate what form of imaging is required. Show the still image of CT scan (Fig. 7.6.2).

## Equipment Required

An equipped SIM suite.
CT head image (Fig. 7.6.2).

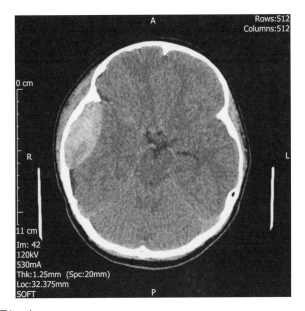

**Figure 7.6.2** CT head.

## Mark Scheme

| | |
|---|---|
| Introduces self and takes role as team leader | |
| Prepares to receive the child: puts out paediatric trauma call and allocates roles | |
| WETFLAG completed appropriately: | |
| • Weight 34 kg (allow reasonable estimate) | |
| • Energy 136 J | |
| • Tube 6/6.5 | |

| | |
|---|---|
| • Fluid 340 ml (trauma) | |
| • Lorazepam 3.4 mg | |
| • Adrenaline 3.4 ml of 1 in 10,000 | |
| • Glucose 68 ml of 10% dextrose | |
| A–E assessment undertaken: | |
| • A: C-spine control and $O_2$ applied | |
| • B: examines chest | |
| • C: obtains IV access and takes bloods | |
| • D: checks GCS, pupils, and blood sugar | |
| • E: exposes child fully, bruising noted. Keeps child warm | |
| Gives IV antibiotics | |
| Considers tetanus status | |
| Discusses the management of the open fracture | |
| **Arranges appropriate analgesia, considers a local anaesthetic block and immobilisation** | |
| **Chooses appropriate imaging** (expect CT head as minimum. Allow pan-CT or selective CT, i.e. to avoid the chest as no clinical indication) | |
| Correctly interprets the CT head: right-sided extradural haemorrhage | |
| Makes a neurosurgical referral and states the intention to prepare the child for theatre | |
| Plans for intubation and neuroprotective measures | |
| Introduces self to parents and checks their identity and knowledge so far | |
| **Explains the course of events and the injuries found** | |
| **Explains what will happen now: theatre required for extradural haemorrhage and open fracture management** | |
| Allows the parents to ask questions, answers appropriately | |
| Gives constructive debrief and thanks the team | |
| Displays effective team leadership skills | |

*NB Up to 2 marks available for actions in bold.*

Total    **/31**

# Learning Points

*Analgesia*

There are various analgesic options in this scenario. Giving analgesia early will allow you to have better control of the situation, as well as being appropriate for a child in distress with multiple injuries. IV or intranasal opiates would be entirely appropriate. IV ketamine at an analgesic dose, such as 0.25–0.5 mg/kg IV, is useful in trauma. Ideally, document the GCS before giving any drugs that can alter the level of consciousness.

*Neuroprotective Measures*

Even in the initial stages, it is worth considering neuroprotection. There are several simple measures in the ED that we can undertake to ensure this:

- Maintain a secure airway and ensure adequate $PaO_2$, aiming for normoxia.
- Optimise venous return from the brain by putting the bed 30° head up (once contraindicating injuries excluded), securing the ETT without tying around the neck and removing the hard collar once safe.
- Maintain an adequate BP, aiming for normotension so as to maintain cerebral perfusion pressure. Correct hypovolaemia promptly.
- Avoid cerebral vasoconstriction by optimising $PaCO_2$, aiming for 35–40 mmHg.
- Use adequate analgesia and sedation. It is important to give adequate analgesia, sedation, and paralysis on induction of anaesthesia and then maintain at an appropriate level.
- Avoid shivering and hypothermia—aim for normothermia.
- Treat seizures promptly.
- Treat hypoglycaemia promptly.

A useful and detailed summary of the evidence and guidelines surrounding traumatic brain injury can be found on the Brain Trauma Foundation website.

# References

https://litfl.com/increased-intracranial-pressure-in-tbi/
https://oxfordmedicine.com/view/10.1093/med/9780198784197.001.0001/med-9780198784197-chapter-8#med-9780198784197-chapter-8-div1-272
https://www.braintrauma.org/coma/guidelines

# 7.7 **Adult Trauma 2**

This is a double station.

## Instructions for Candidate

You receive the following pre-alert: a 40-year-old male is being brought in, having been pulled from a burning car by a passer-by. The car was upside down in a ditch. He has suffered extensive burns and is unconscious on scene. You have five minutes before they arrive to prepare your team. You are working in a burns centre.

## Mark Scheme Breakdown

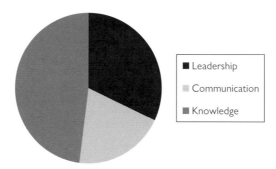

**Figure 7.7.1** Adult trauma 2 mark scheme breakdown.

## Instructions for Actor

*ED Nurses 1 and 2*

You are experienced ED nurses; you are competent and can follow clear instructions.

*Intensive Care SpR*

You are experienced, having completed a trauma fellowship in Australia last year. You are skilled and competent at any necessary procedures. You are currently looking after a patient in the next Resus cubicle and will arrive once the primary survey is complete. When you arrive, you are happy to perform an RSI and will do this promptly and succeed at first attempt. Ask the team leader what they would like for plan A, B, and C before proceeding.

*Surgical SpR*

You have never performed escharotomies before and are reluctant to do so, and attempt to delay the procedure.

# Instructions for Examiner

When requested, the following parameters are available:

- A: patent, there are no visible burns/soot/singeing to airway/face/chest.
- B: RR 20; $SaO_2$ 92% on air, 97% on high flow. Equal chest movement and no obvious bruising or deformity to chest wall. There is equal air entry bilaterally and it is resonant to percussion.
- C: HR 123, BP 92/48. Abdomen is soft. Pelvis is grossly normal. There is an open fracture of the distal tibia. If FAST scan is undertaken, there is no free fluid, pneumothorax, or tamponade.
- D: GCS E1V1M1. Pupils equal, 3 mm. Blood glucose 5.9 mmol/l.
- E: temperature 35.8°C. Extensive haematoma and bruising to right side of head and face. Full-thickness burns to both lower legs circumferentially and palms of hands, estimated at 25%.

There is no evidence of bleeding.

# Equipment Required

An equipped SIM suite.

# Mark Scheme

| | |
|---|---|
| Introduces self and takes the role of team leader | |
| Activates the hospital trauma team | |
| Briefs the team, assigns roles, and discusses any expected issues and the anticipated management plan | |
| Allows the paramedics to hand over and transfer the patient to the ED trolley | |
| Completes the primary survey | |
| Obtains an AMPLE history | |
| Requests high-flow $O_2$ and maintains C-spine protection | |
| Recognises risk to airway and plans for RSI with ITU registrar | |
| States an appropriate airway management plan A, B, and C | |
| Requests a primary survey CXR ± pelvis X-ray | |
| Appropriate volume resuscitation with crystalloid or blood | |
| Recognises likely significant head injury and need for neuroprotective measures | |
| Recognises circumferential full-thickness burns to legs and estimates % burns | |
| Appropriate discussion with surgical SpR to facilitate escharotomies, advises calling consultant/plastics team in | |
| Recognises that once the resuscitation fluids have been given, will need maintenance fluids as per Parkland formula | |

| | |
|---|---|
| Gives IV antibiotics and tetanus coverage | |
| Covers the open fracture with saline-soaked gauze, reduces the fracture, defers application of plaster | |
| Notes temperature and further likelihood of hypothermia. Places Bair Hugger™ | |
| **Has a discussion with team about further management and comes up with a reasonable management plan:**<br>• **Needs urgent escharotomies (theatre or ED?)**<br>• **Needs pan-scan CT if stable (pre- or post-escharotomies?)**<br>• **Needs adequate resuscitation (crystalloid or blood?)**<br>**(Points are awarded on the decision-making, rationale, and quality of discussion with team/surgical SpR)** | |
| Gives constructive debrief and thanks the team | |
| Displays effective team leadership skills | |

*NB Up to 5 marks available for actions in bold.*

Total    /**25**

## Learning Points

Burns in trauma are challenging. A priority must always be the airway and impending failure, even in a seemingly normal airway.

There are multiple other issues to address, and it is challenging to know the correct order. Issues to identify and manage include:

- Fluid management.
- Significant burns which, if circumferential, may impact on the airway or breathing or be a threat to limbs.
- Consider carbon monoxide and cyanide poisoning.
- Keep the patient warm as they will lose heat very quickly.

It is challenging in the trauma scenario to know if volume replacement should be with blood or crystalloid. Once it is confirmed there is no significant bleeding, move to crystalloid, but if in doubt, give blood first.

For patients with >10% body surface area burns, once resuscitation fluids are complete, aim for fluid replacement as per the Parkland formula (fluids = 2–4 ml/kg/% burn). Give 50% in the first eight hours from injury, and then the remaining 50% in the next 16 hours. This is likely to be as the patient leaves the ED for onward care, but it is worth considering in advance. The % burns can be estimated by a variety of methods such as the rule of 9s, the patient's palm, the Lund Browder chart, or the Mersey Burns app.

## Reference

https://www.merseyburns.com

## 7.8 **Adult Trauma 3**

This is a double station.

### Instructions for Candidate

You receive the following pre-alert: a 32-year-old female is being brought in, having been witnessed to jump from a first-storey flat. She appears to be heavily pregnant. She is conscious and distressed. Unfortunately, the signal is lost before you get a complete ATMIST. You have five minutes to prepare.

### Mark Scheme Breakdown

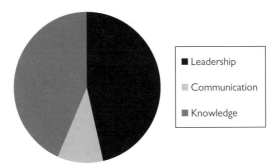

■ Leadership

▨ Communication

▨ Knowledge

**Figure 7.8.1** Adult trauma 3 mark scheme breakdown.

### Instructions for Actor

*ED Nurses 1 and 2*

You are experienced ED nurses. You are competent and can follow clear instructions.

*Surgical SpR*

You have just started your rotation at the trauma centre and have not been involved in many trauma cases yet. You are competent with most procedures and can take direct instructions. You feel very uncomfortable with obstetric trauma. You will call your consultant if asked.

*ITU SpR*

When asked, you are happy to sedate, or perform an RSI on, the patient, although you feel RSI safer but are happy to give some ketamine initially to gain control of the situation whilst preparing for RSI.

*Obstetric SpR*

You feel uncomfortable dealing with trauma in an obstetric patient. You do not feel able to make any decisions but will defer to your consultant when asked. You do not feel there is any uterine rupture and you note a normal foetal HR.

## Instructions for Examiner

When requested, the following parameters are available:

- A: patent, very distressed and combative, confused, and shouting you wish you were dead. Flailing around, unable to maintain C-spine immobilisation.
- B: RR 30; $SaO_2$ 90% on air, 95% on high flow. Equal chest movement and no obvious bruising or deformity to chest wall. There is equal air entry bilaterally and it is resonant to percussion.
- C: HR 133, BP 70/48. Abdomen is gravid, approximately 30 weeks. Pelvis is asymmetrical and binder *in situ*; the left leg appears shorter and there is an open fracture of the right femur.
- If FAST scan is undertaken, there is free fluid around the spleen, but no pneumothorax or tamponade.
- D: GCS E4V4M6. Pupils equal: 4 mm. Blood glucose 4.9 mmol/l.
- E: temperature 36.8°C. Extensive swelling and bleeding in the right thigh/femur.

If the patient is adequately resuscitated with blood products, the patient stabilises. The surgical and obstetric consults arrive, and following a handover and discussion, a decision is made for CT before surgery.

## Equipment Required

An equipped SIM suite.

## Mark Scheme

| | |
|---|---|
| Introduces self and takes role as the team leader | |
| Activates the hospital trauma team. Requests obstetrician in addition | |
| Briefs the team, assigns roles, and discusses expected issues and the management plan | |
| Allows the paramedics to hand over and transfers the patient to ED trolley | |
| Notes gravid uterus and suggests tilting whole trolley to left lateral/manual displacement of the uterus | |
| Completes the primary survey | |
| Asks the obstetric registrar to assess the abdomen also | |
| Recognises haemodynamic instability and activates major haemorrhage protocol, sends two cross-matched samples, including rhesus status | |
| Checks the position of the pelvic binder | |
| Gives tranexamic acid 1 g IV | |
| Obtains an AMPLE history | |
| Requests high-flow $O_2$ and maintains C-spine protection | |
| Requests a primary survey CXR and pelvis X-ray | |

| | |
|---|---|
| Recognises the situation is unmanageable and the need to sedate the patient (Appropriate to proceed to RSI or sedate, e.g. with ketamine to gain control before proceeding) | |
| Initiates volume expansion with blood products (preferably before RSI) | |
| Recognises the patient is too unstable for pan-CT at present but states the ideal direction of travel | |
| Recognises likely significant intra-abdominal, femoral, and pelvic injuries | |
| Covers the open fracture with saline-soaked gauze, reduces the fracture, applies splints | |
| Gives IV antibiotics and tetanus immunisation | |
| Recognises the need for more senior input: calls surgical and obstetric consultants | |
| Provides a succinct handover to the surgical and obstetric consultants | |
| **Has a discussion with the team about further management and comes up with a reasonable management plan:**<br>• **Needs urgent blood products and stabilisation**<br>• **Haemorrhage control: splint femur**<br>• **Considers merits of pan-CT vs damage control surgery, will require general surgery and obstetric input, will need further resuscitation before CT appropriate, but aiming for this**<br>• **Considers role of interventional radiology for splenic injury**<br>**(Points awarded on the decision-making, rationale, and quality of discussion with team)** | |
| Gives constructive debrief and thanks the team | |
| Displays effective team leadership skills | |

*NB Up to 5 marks available for actions in bold.*

Total    **/28**

# Learning Points

This is a complicated case that challenges the candidate to go beyond a simple primary survey. In addition to basic trauma management, the patient is pregnant and so there are also obstetric considerations. There are complex decisions to be made, which requires significant situational awareness and good communication skills with the whole team, and recognition of the level of expertise of the team members.

The minutes before the patient arrives are crucial. Use them to anticipate the injuries and complications, based on the pre-alert information. Discuss the likely procedures and pathways with the team, including the specialties, and prepare any equipment that may be needed.

It is important to do the simple things well—a thorough primary survey, correcting the abnormalities as they are found; optimising the position for the gravid patient; and providing adequate analgesia.

Practise until there is fluency in your trauma management, which will allow you the headspace to focus on the more complex tasks and decision-making.

# Chapter 8 **Psychiatry Scenarios**

# The Psychiatry Station

It is almost guaranteed that you will have a mental health station in the FRCEM OSCE, so make sure you are comfortable with, and competent at, taking a psychiatric history. You should be able to do a risk assessment and undertake a capacity assessment fluently. Familiarise yourself with the Mental Capacity Act and the various Mental Health Acts, and know when each should apply. The scenarios within this chapter will give you the opportunity to practise these skills and apply the relevant assessment tools or Acts.

# 8.1 Deliberate Self-Harm

## Instructions for Candidate

A 17-year-old girl has been brought to the ED after she cut her wrists with a pair of scissors. The wounds are superficial and have already been dressed. Please take a focused history and assess the patient's risk and capacity.

## Mark Scheme Breakdown

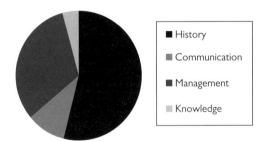

- History
- Communication
- Management
- Knowledge

**Figure 8.1.1** Deliberate self-harm mark scheme breakdown.

## Instructions for Actor

You are a 17-year-old girl. You have attended today after cutting your wrists with a pair of scissors. You cut with the intention of taking your life but became scared and changed your mind as it hurt more than you had expected. A friend brought you to the ED, but they have gone to make a phone call. You remain upset after splitting up with your boyfriend. It is the first time you have done this and although it was impulsive, you remain suicidal. You have decided to jump off the Tamar bridge once you leave the ED. You refuse to stay and see the psychiatry team and will abscond from the ED, given the chance.

## Instructions for Examiner

Observation only. At one minute before the end of the OSCE, prompt the candidate for their summary. Ask for their evaluation on the patient's risk and capacity.

## Equipment Required

None.

## Mark Scheme

| | |
|---|---|
| Introduces self to the patient | |
| Confirms the patient is currently safe and her injuries addressed | |
| Asks an open question to assess the presenting complaint | |
| Establishes details: | |
| • What injuries occurred and how they were sustained | |
| • Whether it was planned or impulsive | |
| • What she thought would happen with injury. Was there suicidal intent? | |
| • Final acts, e.g. a suicide note, sorting out financial affairs | |
| • How she was discovered | |
| • Alcohol and drug use | |
| • Any precipitating events | |
| • Suicidal ideation now? Regretful? | |
| Performs a risk assessment: SADPERSON or gestalt | |
| Asks about sleep, appetite, and enjoyment | |
| Past medical history | |
| Past psychiatric history | |
| Drug history | |
| Social history: friends/family she can talk to? How is work/home affected? | |
| Forensic history | |
| Assesses capacity: | |
| • Establishes if there is impairment of the mind/brain | |
| • Confirms the patient understands | |
| • Establishes if the patient can weigh up the risks and benefits | |
| • Establishes if she can retain the information | |
| • Establishes if the patient can communicate her decision | |
| States needs a mental state examination | |
| Summarises: high risk, has capacity | |

| Discusses the management: psychiatric assessment for full mental health assessment (MHA) | |
|---|---|
| Establishes a good rapport with the patient | |
| Explains and negotiates with patient to stay | |

Total    **/28**

# Learning Points

*The Mental Capacity Act (MCA) 2005*

The MCA details a two-stage test of capacity:

1. Does the person have an impairment or a disturbance in the functioning of their mind or brain? This can include, for example, conditions associated with mental illness, concussion, or symptoms of drug or alcohol abuse.
2. Does the impairment or disturbance mean that the person is unable to make a specific decision when they need to? You should offer all appropriate and practical support to achieve this before applying this stage of the test.

*Functional Tests of Capacity*

To make a decision, a person should be able to:

- Understand the decision to be made and the information provided about the decision. The consequences of making a decision must be included in the information given.
- Retain the information: a person should be able to retain the information given for long enough to make the decision. If information can only be retained for short periods of time, it should not automatically be assumed that the person lacks capacity. Notebooks, for example, could be used to record information which may help a person to retain it.
- Use that information in making the decision: a person should be able to weigh up the pros and cons of making the decision.
- Communicate their decision: if a person cannot communicate their decision; for example, if they are in a coma, the Act specifies that they should be treated as if they lack capacity. You should make all efforts to help the person communicate their decision before deciding they cannot.

## 8.2 **Opiate Overdose**

### Instructions for Candidate

A 78-year-old woman has been brought to the ED after she was found to be drowsy, with a reduced RR and pinpoint pupils. The paramedics gave her naloxone and she is now alert, with normal vital signs. Please take a focused history and assess the patient's capacity.

### Mark Scheme Breakdown

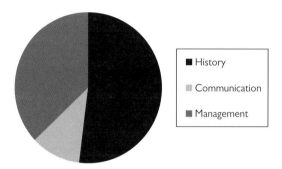

- History
- Communication
- Management

**Figure 8.2.1** Opiate overdose mark scheme breakdown.

### Instructions for Actor

You are a 78-year-old lady. You are very tearful; your husband died six months ago and you have been recently diagnosed with metastatic lung cancer. You had placed all your opiate patches on yourself with the intention of drifting off to sleep and never waking up. You are disappointed as your neighbour raised the alarm when they noted the curtains were still closed at midday. You had left notes and a copy of your will for your two sons on the kitchen table.

You live alone and have a medical history that includes hypertension, atrial fibrillation, COPD, and lung cancer. You take ramipril, apixaban, tiotropium, salbutamol, bisoprolol, co-codamol, and buprenorphine (Transtec®) patches. You have no allergies. You are independent and an ex-smoker, and drink minimal alcohol. You are a retired dentist and are orientated in time, place, and person.

You have capacity when assessed. However, you remain intent on taking your own life but agree to an assessment by the Mental Health team.

### Instructions for Examiner

Observation only. At one minute before the end of the OSCE, prompt the candidate for their summary and ask for their evaluation of the patient's capacity.

# Equipment Required

None.

# Mark Scheme

| | |
|---|---|
| Introduces self to the patient | |
| Checks the patient is safe and patches removed | |
| Asks an open question to assess the presenting complaint | |
| Establishes details: | |
| • Planned or impulsive | |
| • Intention | |
| • Final acts, e.g. suicide note, sorting financial affairs | |
| • How she was discovered | |
| • Alcohol and drug use | |
| • Precipitant | |
| • Suicidal ideation now | |
| Performs a risk assessment: SADPERSON or gestalt | |
| Asks about biological symptoms of depression | |
| Past medical history | |
| Past psychiatric history | |
| Drug history | |
| Social history | |
| Forensic history | |
| Assesses capacity: | |
| • Establishes if there is impairment of the mind/brain | |
| • Confirms the patient understands | |
| • Establishes if the patient can weigh up the risks and benefits | |
| • Establishes if the patient can retain the information | |
| • Establishes if the patient can communicate her decision | |
| States the patient will need a mental state examination | |

| | |
|---|---|
| Summarises: high risk, has capacity | |
| Provides an explanation to the patient | |
| Sensitively negotiates with the patient to stay to be assessed by the Mental Health team | |
| Discusses the plan: psychiatric assessment | |

Total    **/27**

## Learning Points

It is no longer recommended that we make decisions on risk and decide to discharge patients based on a specific score such as the SAD PERSONS scale (Table 8.2.1) or similar tool. However, it still serves as a useful scale to guide an assessment of risk and prompt specific questions in the history. Frequently, we ask psychiatry liaison to assess these patients and make the risk assessment, which also facilitates the arrangement of outpatient follow-up. It is helpful to have an assessment of risk to facilitate referral of these patients and to allow psychiatry to triage their patients.

**Table 8.2.1** Modified SAD PERSONS scale

| | Score |
|---|---|
| Male sex | 1 |
| Age <19 or >45 years | 1 |
| Depression or hopelessness | 2 |
| Previous suicide attempts or psychiatric care | 1 |
| Excessive alcohol or drug use | 1 |
| Rational thinking loss (psychotic or organic illness) | 2 |
| Separated, widowed, or divorced | 1 |
| Organised or serious attempt | 2 |
| No social support | 1 |
| Stated future intent (determined to repeat or ambivalent) | 2 |

# 8.3 **Mental State Examination**

## Instructions for Candidate

A 42-year-old woman has been brought to the ED after being found behaving oddly in the street. Please take a history and present your findings to the examiner.

## Mark Scheme Breakdown

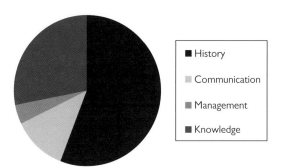

**Figure 8.3.1** Mental state examination mark scheme breakdown.

## Instructions for Actor

You are a 42-year-old lady, you have been brought here by paramedics after they were called when you were found in the street. You had been trying to climb up a monument in the city centre and shouting 'all hail the new princess'. You are extremely talkative with pressure of speech. You believe you have just discovered that you are a member of the Royal family and have resigned from your job (as an office cleaner). You desperately want to get to London to claim the throne and to go to Harrods to buy some new clothes suitable for a new princess.

You have no previous medical or psychiatric history. You take no medication and have no allergies. No forensic history. You drink a bottle of wine a week and deny any illicit drug use. You live alone in a one-bedroomed flat. You are orientated in time, place, and person but lack insight into your condition.

## Instructions for Examiner

Observation only. At one minute before the end of the OSCE, prompt the candidate for their summary and mental state examination findings if they have not done so already.

## Equipment Required

None.

## Mark Scheme

| | |
|---|---|
| Introduces self to the patient | |
| Asks an open question to assess the presenting complaint | |
| Establishes further details: | |
| • Explores the history—what happened today | |
| • Grandiose ideas | |
| • Excessive spending | |
| • Biological symptoms | |
| • Hallucinations | |
| • Self-harm and suicidal ideation | |
| • Alcohol and drug use | |
| • Precipitants | |
| Past medical history | |
| Past psychiatric history, including previous MHA | |
| Drug history | |
| Social history | |
| Forensic history | |
| Undertakes and then presents the mental state examination | |
| Comments on: | |
| • Appearance and behaviour | |
| • Speech | |
| • Mood and affect | |
| • Thought | |
| • Perceptions | |
| • Cognition | |
| • Insight | |
| Sensitively explains the findings and the plan to the patient | |
| Closes the station appropriately and thanks the patient | |

Total    /**25**

## Learning Points

This is a challenging station as there is a lot to cover within the time frame, especially as these patients are frequently distracting and talkative. You need to get the specifics of what happened, as well as obtain a full mental state examination and medical history. You will then need to explain your concerns and the plan to the patient. You may be asked to present your findings and management plan to the examiner.

A full psychiatric history is often taken by psychiatric liaison rather than us, but there is no reason why you should not take one. Severe psychiatric illness occurs more commonly in the exam than in the ED. If you get the opportunity to assess a patient with mania or psychosis, make sure you work through a full mental state examination and experience the challenges it can pose.

## 8.4 **Paracetamol Overdose**

### Instructions for Candidate

A 28-year-old woman has been brought to the ED after taking an overdose of 48 tablets of paracetamol 500 mg. Her 4-hour paracetamol level has just been phoned through from the lab and is 129 mg/l. She wants to leave the ED. Please take a focused history and assess the patient's capacity.

### Mark Scheme Breakdown

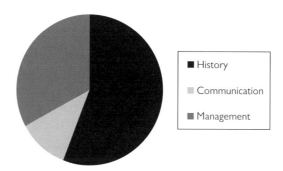

**Figure 8.4.1** Paracetamol overdose mark scheme breakdown.

### Instructions for Actor

You are a 28-year-old lady, and you have taken an overdose of 48 paracetamol tablets about six hours ago (not with alcohol). It was impulsive after an argument with your partner. You want to die to spite him. You had posted a message on social media after the overdose and a concerned friend raised the alarm and called an ambulance. You agreed to have blood tests, but now you want to leave the department.

You have no formal mental health diagnosis but have had repeated attendances to ED with overdoses and deliberate self-harm (DSH). You take no medication and have no allergies. There is no forensic history. You drink a bottle of vodka a week and smoke 15 cigarettes a day, with occasional cannabis use.

You live with your partner and are unemployed. If the candidate gains a rapport and explains the risks of leaving and not having treatment, then you agree to stay. If they do not, you become difficult and tearful.

### Instructions for Examiner

Observation only. At one minute before the end of the OSCE, prompt the candidate for their summary and ask for their evaluation of the patient's capacity.

### Equipment Required

None.

# Mark Scheme

| | |
|---|---|
| Introduces self to the patient | |
| Checks the patient is currently safe | |
| Asks an open question to assess the presenting complaint | |
| Establishes further details: | |
| • Planned/impulsive | |
| • What did the patient think would happen with that many tablets? Was there suicidal intent? | |
| • Regret? | |
| • Final acts, e.g. suicide note, sorting financial affairs | |
| • How they were discovered | |
| • Alcohol and drug use | |
| • Any precipitating events | |
| • Suicidal ideation now? | |
| Performs risk assessment: SAD PERSONS or gestalt | |
| Asks about biological symptoms of depression | |
| Past medical history | |
| Past psychiatric history | |
| Drug history | |
| Social history | |
| Forensic history | |
| Assesses capacity: | |
| • Establishes/states no impairment of mind/brain | |
| • Confirms the patient understands | |
| • Establishes if the patient can weigh up the risks and benefits | |
| • Establishes if the patient can retain the information | |
| • Establishes if the patient can communicate her decision | |
| Explains the concerns and the management plan to the patient | |
| Gains rapport and negotiates with the patient to stay | |
| States the patient needs a formal mental state examination and psychiatric evaluation/MHA | |
| Summarises: high risk, has capacity | |

Total    /**27**

## Learning Points

This can be a tricky station with regard to time management as there is a lot of material to cover. The key elements of the station are:

- Checking patient safety—do they need medical treatment?
- Taking a history of events.
- Completing a medical history, and social, forensic, and past medical history, etc.
- Making a risk assessment.
- Assessing capacity.

To achieve all of this, you need to establish a good rapport early on and direct the conversation effectively.

## 8.5 **Assessment of a Confused Patient**

### Instructions for Candidate

Mrs Smith has brought in her mother aged 75 years who is acutely confused. Please perform a cognitive assessment and explain the next steps in her management.

### Mark Scheme Breakdown

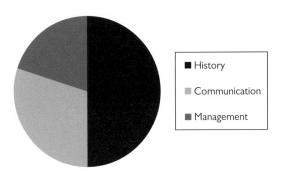

**Figure 8.5.1** Assessment of a confused patient mark scheme breakdown.

### Instructions for Actor

*Mrs Smith*

You are very worried about your mother; she was completely orientated yesterday, but today she is muddled. You are keen to know what is going to happen next and if she will get better. You are very concerned this means that she has dementia.

*Elderly Mother*

Your name is Elsie. You do not know why you are here and why people are fussing. You just want to go home to have a cup of tea and watch East Enders.

You are very confused. You do not know the correct year/season/month/day or time but guess an answer for each. You know in which country and town you are, but you are not able to clarify further. You are able to repeat the names of two of the three objects. You make no effort when asked to perform simple calculations. You can recall one of the previous three objects. You can name the items when asked. You fail to repeat a specified sentence. You can obey simple instructions and, when asked to write a sentence, you just sign your name. You are unable to copy a diagram.

### Instructions for Examiner

Observation only.

# Equipment Required

Props for the assessment, e.g. ball, apple, comb, pen, and a piece of paper.

# Mark Scheme

| | |
|---|---|
| Introduces self to the patient and her relative | |
| Establishes who the relative is and elicits their concerns | |
| Explains the need to ask a series of questions as part of the assessment | |
| Tests orientation in time | |
| Tests orientation in place | |
| Tests registration of new information | |
| Tests attention and calculation | |
| Tests recall | |
| Tests repetition | |
| Tests the patient's ability to perform commands | |
| Tests the patient's ability to read and write | |
| Has a patient and reassuring manner and asks questions at an appropriate pace | |
| Correctly scores the patient and grades the severity | |
| Explains further management of the case when asked by the relative: | |
| • Initial investigations—ECG, urine dip, bloods, CT head, etc. | |
| • Medication review | |
| • Review by the frailty team | |
| Answers questions regarding dementia and delirium appropriately and in a reassuring manner | |
| Closes the consultation appropriately | |

Total    /**18**

# Learning Points

The MMSE is a commonly used assessment of cognition and, although widely available, is subject to copyright. Nonetheless, it is worth familiarising yourself with the MMSE. Know what the components are and practise the examination until it becomes fluent. This will allow you to focus on building a rapport with the patient and on formulating a sensible management plan.

# 8.6 **Alcohol History**

## Instructions for Candidate

It is 9 a.m., and a nurse practitioner has just treated a lady's wound but is concerned she smells strongly of alcohol and would like you to review her before she leaves the ED. Please take a focused alcohol history from this patient and then advise her of further management.

## Mark Scheme Breakdown

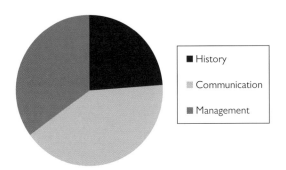

**Figure 8.6.1** Alcohol history mark scheme breakdown.

## Instructions for Actor

You are a 42-year-old estate agent and have attended the ED this morning after falling and cutting your arm yesterday evening on a night out. The wound has been cleaned and closed by the ENP already.

When asked about alcohol, you are cagey but answer honestly if the candidate asks in an appropriate and non-judgemental way. You drink most days and will normally consume a bottle of wine each evening. The most you would ever drink in one day is two bottles of wine. Your attendance in the ED is alcohol-related as you had consumed two cocktails and then four large glasses of wine with work friends prior to the fall.

You do not want to be referred to any alcohol services as you think this is normal 'social' drinking. You want to leave to go to work as you have several house viewings booked. You become angry and then tearful when the candidate gives you advice. You are particularly worried about losing your job as you need to drive to get to viewings.

## Instructions for Examiner

Observation only.

## Equipment Required

None.

## Mark Scheme

| | |
|---|---|
| Introduces self to the patient | |
| Checks the patient is comfortable | |
| Explains the ENP wanted a review and that concerns were raised | |
| Obtains a brief alcohol history, e.g. Paddington Alcohol Test (PAT), Alcohol Use Disorders Identification Test (AUDIT-C), or Fast Alcohol Screening Test (FAST) | |
| Asks about social history and employment | |
| Past medical history | |
| Drug history | |
| Suggests she may still be over the driving limit and should not drive to work | |
| Advises she would be criminally responsible if she were to drive and crash, and would not be insured | |
| Explains concerns: | |
| • Drinking above safe recommended amounts | |
| • Today's attendance is alcohol-related | |
| • Concerned for future escalation | |
| • Affecting her health and impact on life | |
| Advises the patient to cut down and explains why | |
| Offers referral to alcohol support team | |
| Establishes good rapport and offers sensitive explanations | |
| Closes appropriately | |

Total    /**17**

## Learning Points

The General Medical Council (GMC)'s *Good Medical Practice*, the DVLA's *Assessing Fitness to Drive*, and the RCEM's *Alcohol Toolkit* documents are all relevant to this case and worth reading and referring to.

## References

https://www.gmc-uk.org/ethical-guidance/ethical-guidance-for-doctors/good-medical-practice

https://assets.publishing.service.gov.uk/government/uploads/system/uploads/attachment_data/file/783444/assessing-fitness-to-drive-a-guide-for-medical-professionals.pdf

https://www.rcem.ac.uk/docs/College%20Guidelines/5z24.%20Alcohol%20toolkit%20(June%202015).pdf

Patterson et al, (1983), Evaluation of suicidal patients: The SAD PERSONS scale, Elsevier, Psychosomatics. 24, 4, pg7.

# Chapter 9 **Management Scenarios**

# The Management Station

In the more recent cohorts of the FRCEM OSCE, there have been scenarios that are designed to test your management skills. Try to gain experience in your own department answering complaints and dealing with serious incidents, as well as gaining the tools to manage a busy and crowded department. Good communication is integral to good management. It is a skill to know when to be concise and process lots of information, and when to be more empathetic and supportive, all whilst making important management decisions. This chapter includes clinically useful examples to work through.

# 9.1 **Ambulance Corridor Triage**

## Instructions for Candidate

The nurse in charge of the ED has asked you to help prioritise the management of the patients currently queuing in the ambulance corridor. You have one Resus bed available and one Majors cubicle; however, there are eight patients waiting.

## Mark Scheme Breakdown

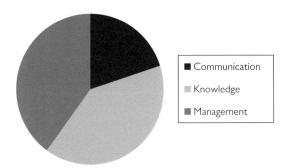

**Figure 9.1.1** Ambulance corridor triage mark scheme breakdown.

## Instructions for Actor

*ED Nurse in Charge*

You are nearly at the end of a very busy shift and are feeling overwhelmed. You have asked the senior ED trainee to help safely triage the ambulance queue but know the resources are limited. The information in brackets is available if the candidate specifically asks.

The ambulance corridor has the following patients:

1. A 25-year-old female who has taken a paracetamol overdose—(32 × 500 mg, five hours ago), frequent attender, tends to abscond, currently has capacity.
2. A 34-year-old male who sustained laceration to scalp after falling—intoxicated, (GCS 14/15), no other NICE criteria for CT head, wound needs sutures.
3. A 62-year-old male with chest pain—nil acute on prehospital ECG, observations fine, and looks well, but had (ST-elevation myocardial infarction (STEMI) five months ago).
4. An 82-year-old male with shortened and externally rotated right leg—slipped on wet floor, no other injuries, had (IV opiates with crew), observations stable.
5. A 73-year-old female with shortness of breath and high temperature—(observations: RR 32, HR 136, BP 83/45, temperature 39.1°C). Past medical history: hypertension (HTN). Looks very unwell.
6. A 38-year-old female with ankle injury—obvious deformity, in vacuum splint, pulses present, and no critical skin. Fell down full flight of stairs. (Also has lumbar back pain and graze to head).

7. A 20-month-old boy with febrile convulsion—first seizure, lasted one minute, temperature 38.8°C, Paediatric Early Warning Score (PEWS) 4, clingy but alert.

8. A 14-year-old girl with abdominal pain, seen by GP a week earlier and started on antibiotics for presumed UTI—HR 132, otherwise normal observations.

## Instructions for Examiner

Observation only.

## Equipment Required

None.

## Mark Scheme

| | |
|---|---|
| Introduces self to the nurse in charge | |
| Checks what she needs help with | |
| Recognises she is task-overloaded, offers to help | |
| Deals effectively with each patient in turn | |
| Patient 1: | |
| • Clarifies what was taken, how much, and when | |
| • Assesses absconding risk/capacity | |
| • Checks vital signs | |
| • Suggests the patient needs bloods now | |
| • Documents the patient's description and allocates to a visible area | |
| Patient 2: | |
| • Checks the GCS | |
| • Checks vital signs | |
| • Assesses capacity | |
| • Asks about head injury red flags | |
| • Suggests a safe management plan | |
| Patient 3: | |
| • Checks vital signs | |
| • Enquires about ECG changes | |
| • Ensures analgesia is offered | |

| | |
|---|---|
| • Offers to review the patient | |
| • Suggests a safe management plan | |
| Patient 4: | |
| • Asks about the mechanism of injury and the cause for the fall | |
| • Asks about other injuries and ensures analgesia is given | |
| • Checks vital signs | |
| • Suggests investigations (X-ray, bloods, ECG) | |
| • Suggests a fast-track referral to orthopaedics | |
| Patient 5: | |
| • Checks vital signs | |
| • Offers to quickly review the patient | |
| • Suggests moving the patient to the Resus bay | |
| • Indicates will send a doctor in to see the patient | |
| • Prescribes antibiotics, IV fluids, and $O_2$ | |
| Patient 6: | |
| • Asks about deformity, open or closed injury, critical skin, and pulses | |
| • Asks about the mechanism and other injuries | |
| • Ensures analgesia is given | |
| • Checks vital signs | |
| • Escalates appropriately (e.g. trauma call on hearing it was a fall down a full flight of stairs) | |
| Patient 7: | |
| • Asks about the patient's conscious level | |
| • Checks the vital signs or PEWS | |
| • Asks about the duration of the seizure | |
| • Asks whether the seizure self-terminated or required drugs/antipyretics | |
| • Suggests streaming to paediatrics | |
| Patient 8: | |
| • Suggests a review of the patient | |
| • Checks the vital signs | |
| • Requests a urine dip and pregnancy test | |

| | |
|---|---|
| • Requests blood tests | |
| • Considers whether the patient is well enough for urgent care or primary care streaming | |
| Demonstrates good communication and decision-making skills with the nurse in charge | |
| Performs a welfare check on the nurse in charge: checks staffing and breaks | |
| Suggests escalation to the on-call manager, consultant at home, and other teams | |
| Summarises and closes appropriately | |

Total    /**48**

## Learning Points

This station allows you to demonstrate a large amount of clinical knowledge and senior decision-making. The key to doing well in this station is to recognise that as well as the obvious patient safety factors, there is a staff welfare and communication element. You need to focus on the vital clinical elements to ensure each patient is safe and then move on swiftly as this station goes very quickly. You must hone in on the relevant information to enable you to make a management decision that keeps the department safe. The other key element is to recognise your stressed and overstretched nursing colleague and offer some suggestions to help, whilst communicating effectively and empathetically.

# 9.2 **Departmental Handover**

## Instructions for Candidate

It is 8 a.m. handover and you are the oncoming consultant in charge. Please safely lead the handover meeting, including the allocation of your staff.

- In Majors: there are five patients who have been seen by the night team and 11 waiting to be seen.
- In Minors/Urgent Care: there are eight patients waiting to be seen.
- Staffing: you plus one clinical decision ward consultant, two registrars, two SHOs (one is a locum), and two nurse practitioners.

## Mark Scheme Breakdown

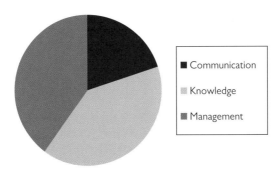

**Figure 9.2.1** Handover mark scheme breakdown.

## Instructions for Actor

*Night Registrar (DF)*

You are tired after a busy shift and are keen to get home. You provide the following information, with the details in brackets if asked specifically:

If asked, there is a trauma patient on their way in—a 64-year-old motorcyclist vs car. Suspected flail chest and pelvic injuries. Tachycardic at 105, but other vital signs are normal range. Estimated time of arrival (ETA) 15 minutes.

Angela Hopkins: polypharmacy overdose awaiting bed—drugs taken: paracetamol, naproxen, sertraline, and diazepam at 7 p.m. Bloods, including paracetamol levels, are fine. She has been referred to the mental health team. She has capacity if she chooses to leave and is at low/ moderate risk of further suicidal attempts.

Iris Pengelly: urosepsis awaiting medical bed—she has had co-amoxiclav and the full sepsis bundle. Not for treatment escalation, and medical SpR and the patient's family are all aware.

Stuart Lewis: head injury awaiting CT report—brief loss of consciousness, vomited twice and is on rivaroxaban. GCS 15 throughout. Home if normal.

If asked about the unseen patients—offer that Colin McCardle should have an early review as has sepsis markers and is an IVDU.

*Night SHO (AB)*

You saw Brett Jones; he is a regular attender who came in intoxicated. He has been left to sleep it off. (If asked, you did not examine him as he always comes in like this. GCS was 'about 10' and you are unsure if he had any signs of injury.)

*Night SHO (MC)*

You saw Marjorie Bailey who is being treated as ACS and is awaiting a cardiology bed (ECG: dynamic inferolateral changes, troponin is outstanding, and you have asked cardiology to review urgently).

*Locum SHO 1*

On F3 year. Worked here several times before and has all appropriate logins.

## Instructions for Examiner

Observation only.

## Equipment Required

Screenshot of patients in department (Table 9.2.1).

**Table 9.2.1** Screenshot of patients in the department.

| Name | Age (years) | Presenting complaint | Doctor | Time (minutes) |
|---|---|---|---|---|
| Angela Hopkins | 36 | Mixed overdose | DF | 344 |
| Brett Jones | 44 | Intoxicated | AB | 312 |
| Iris Pengelly | 92 | Urosepsis | DF | 303 |
| Stuart Lewis | 68 | Head injury | AB | 298 |
| Marjorie Bailey | 68 | Chest pain | MC | 245 |
| Donald Carter | 81 | Haematemesis | | 180 |
| Dorothy Miller | 78 | Acute confusion | | 127 |
| Piotr Kowalski | 67 | Social concerns | | 119 |
| Charlene Smith | 24 | Abdominal pain | | 110 |
| Richard Ackerman | 79 | Short of breath | | 99 |
| Ida Coombes | 88 | Fall | | 89 |
| Rohit Patel | 52 | Chest pain | | 87 |
| Roberto Constanti | 33 | Mental health | | 77 |
| James Sampson | 67 | Unable to urinate | | 70 |
| Colin McCardle | 40 | Groin abscess | | 51 |
| Amy Swains | 28 | Bleeding in pregnancy | | 22 |

# Mark Scheme

| | |
|---|---|
| Introduces self to the team | |
| Checks all staff are present and OK | |
| Thanks the night team for their work | |
| Checks if there were any issues overnight with equipment or teams | |
| Enquires about absconding patients or urgent items to follow up | |
| Checks if there are urgent cases or traumas inbound | |
| Allocates either the SpR or clinical decision ward consultant to take the inbound trauma | |
| Allocates staff to Majors/Minors | |
| Checks if there are any learning needs for the trainees | |
| Clarifies locum SHO experience: background/worked in department before/logins required | |
| Hands over each patient in turn safely | |
| Patient 1 (AH): | |
| • Checks what drugs were taken | |
| • Checks assessments of capacity and risk were made, and a referral requested | |
| • Checks bloods and whether there are any outstanding jobs | |
| Patient 2 (B): | |
| • Asks if a head injury was sustained | |
| • Confirms the GCS | |
| • Checks the social situation | |
| Patient 3 (IP): | |
| • Checks the current vital signs | |
| • Checks that antibiotics were given and asks if any jobs are outstanding | |
| • Asks if escalation is appropriate and whether the family are aware of the admission | |
| Patient 4 (SL): | |
| • Asks if there are any head injury red flags | |

| | |
|---|---|
| • Checks the GCS | |
| • Asks about imaging results and the onward plan | |
| Patient 5 (MB): | |
| • Enquires about ECG changes | |
| • Checks the troponin level | |
| • Confirms a cardiology referral was made | |
| Gives appropriate feedback to the SHO on the assessment of intoxicated patients and head injuries in a sensitive and educational manner | |
| Thanks and discharges the night team and allocates roles to day team members | |
| Suggests an announcement to the patients to in waiting room to apologise for long waits | |
| Suggests a safety round of vital signs and drugs | |

Total    /**30**

## Learning Points

This is a great station as it is a true reflection of a day at work. Practise doing this for real before the exam. You need to recognise that you have tired night staff who may not divulge all the information to you unless specifically asked. As in real life, we sometimes need to review patients from the end of a shift with a fresh pair of eyes. It is crucial to obtain key clinical information to ensure patient safety is maintained for handed-over patients. This should be done in a manner that is neither judgemental nor critical of the night team. Where appropriate, offer educational points to the team.

## 9.3 **Missed Fracture**

### Instructions for Candidate

You have been asked to see Mrs Johns, a 45-year-old lady who fell two days ago and was seen in the ED by one of the F2 doctors. She was discharged with a soft tissue injury and no follow-up was arranged. Her X-ray is provided.

### Mark Scheme Breakdown

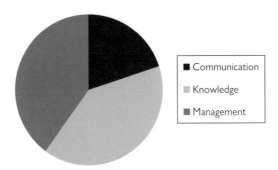

**Figure 9.3.1** Missed fracture mark scheme breakdown.

### Instructions for Actor

*Mrs Johns*

You fell whilst getting off a bus two days ago and injured your knee. You are unable to put any weight on it and it has become more swollen and painful since you were seen. You were told it was a soft tissue injury and advised to take over-the-counter pain relief and given crutches. If the candidate is apologetic and provides a good explanation and ongoing management, you are relieved and calm. If the news is broken badly, you become angry and want to put in a formal complaint about the junior doctor and the missed fracture.

### Instructions for Examiner

Observation only.

# Equipment Required

X-rays provided (Figs. 9.3.2 and 9.3.3).

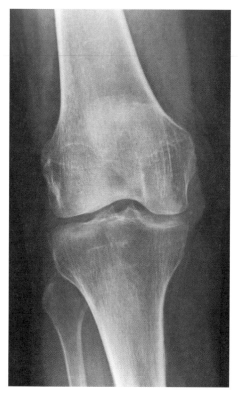

**Figure 9.3.2** AP knee X-ray.

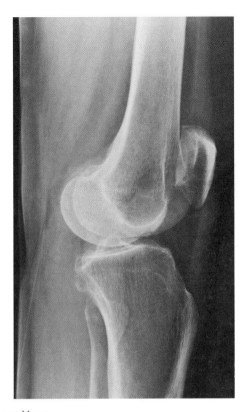

**Figure 9.3.3** Lateral knee X-ray.

Reproduced from Fig 91.1 and Fig 91.2, from Case 91, in Musculoskeletal Imaging Cases, by Mark W. Anderson and Stacy E. Smith, Oxford University Press ISBN: 9780195394375.

## Mark Scheme

| | |
|---|---|
| Introduces self to the patient | |
| Offers analgesia | |
| Asks an open question to assess the presenting complaint | |
| Clarifies the history of events | |
| Correctly recognises a tibial plateau fracture from the X-rays | |
| Apologises for the missed diagnosis | |
| Uses the X-ray images to demonstrate the fracture to the patient | |
| Explains will organise a referral to orthopaedics | |
| Explains the need for CT and consideration of operative management or knee brace | |

| | |
|---|---|
| States will give feedback to the junior doctor in question | |
| Suggests will arrange teaching sessions for all the junior doctors in ED | |
| Ensures the patient understands the plan from here | |
| Offers details for PALS and explains how to submit a formal complaint | |
| Closes the conversation | |

Total    /**14**

## Learning Points

This is essentially a communication station. However, for it to go well, you need to be well informed on hospital complaint policies and offer the patient the option to complain. Familiarise yourself with your hospital's complaint procedure.

It is fine to admit a mistake was made or an injury was missed. This can be done in a non-accusatory way, explaining that fractures are sometimes hard to see and can be missed. Indeed, that is why we have the double-check systems in place once X-rays are reported. Diffusing the situation is paramount—it is important not to be dragged into an argument. An apology goes a long way. Show empathy and understanding for the distress they may have incurred.

## 9.4 **Serious Incident Management**

### Instructions for Candidate

You are the incoming consultant and are met by the nurse in charge to hear that the night ST3 doctor inserted a chest drain into the wrong side of a patient's chest. Please advise the nurse what needs to be done now.

### Mark Scheme Breakdown

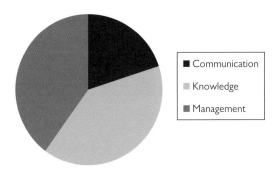

**Figure 9.4.1** Serious incident mark scheme breakdown.

### Instructions for Actor

*Staff Nurse*

You were the sister in charge overnight and are reporting that the ST3 doctor inserted a Seldinger chest drain into the wrong side. The patient had initially been seen by a different doctor and diagnosed with a secondary pneumothorax and the ST3 was asked to insert the drain. No checklist was used, but formal consent was documented. When she realised what had happened, she was mortified, explained what had happened to the patient, and has now gone to the staff room in tears. The patient is still in Resus with his family but is not immediately compromised.

### Instructions for Examiner

Observation only.

### Equipment Required

None.

## Mark Scheme

| | |
|---|---|
| Introduces self to the nurse and clarifies her concern | |
| Checks the patient is safe, confirms the patient still needs the chest drain | |
| Arranges immediate ongoing care: further imaging/bilateral chest drains | |
| States will speak to the patient and the family (apology/duty of candour) | |
| States will need to secure the notes and imaging and make copies | |
| States will get statements from all the staff involved | |
| States will need to submit a DATIX/incident form | |
| Considered a never event, so will need full investigation | |
| Checks the ST3 is OK, likely too upset to work and needs to go home | |
| Ascertains when the ST3 doctor is next due to work | |
| Suggests extra support for the ST3 on the next shift | |
| Asks if this is the first incident for ST3 | |
| States will inform her supervisor for additional support | |
| Considers the impact on immediate staffing (e.g. next night shift) | |
| Highlights the event to the clinical governance lead and medical director | |
| Considers future education, e.g. guideline, introduction of safety checklist | |
| Asks if there are any further questions and closes discussion | |

Total    /**17**

## Learning Points

The website under References is a useful resource for reading about serious incidents, never events, and patient safety issues.

## References

https://www.england.nhs.uk/patient-safety/serious-incident-framework/

## 9.5 **Major Incident Management**

### Instructions for Candidate

Please liaise with the ED sister who has just taken an emergency telephone call regarding a major incident. She has not been involved in a major incident before and has some questions.

### Mark Scheme Breakdown

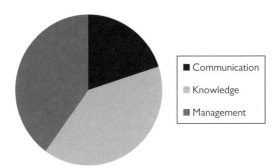

**Figure 9.5.1** Major incident mark scheme breakdown.

### Instructions for Actor

You are a newly appointed junior ED sister and have not been involved with a major incident before. You have just taken a red phone call from ambulance control stating a major incident has been declared. You have not heard of 'METHANE', but you have some information. A major incident has been declared. A 3-vehicle pile-up on the motorway occurred 40 minutes ago. An unknown chemical has leaked from a lorry, so extrication has been slow. You are unsure how many casualties there are or what the expected time of arrival is, but you know there has been one fatality on scene. You want to discuss the process now of how to ready the department, who to call, and what your role is.

### Equipment Required

None.

### Mark Scheme

| | |
|---|---|
| Introduces self to the nurse | |
| Establishes previous experience of running the department and major incident involvement | |
| Asks the nurse if she has specific concerns | |

| | |
|---|---|
| Clarifies the details received from METHANE: | |
| • M: Major incident declared or standby | |
| • E: Exact location of the incident | |
| • T: Time of the incident | |
| • H: Hazards present | |
| • A: Access to the scene | |
| • N: Number and severity of casualties | |
| • E: Emergency services on scene | |
| Discusses the process for readying the department: | |
| • Phones ambulance control and confirms genuine if concerned | |
| • Activates the major incident cascade via switch | |
| • Informs the lead consultant/nurse | |
| • Allocates an administrator to get staff mobile numbers and to call in extra staff (remind them they will need ID to get in) | |
| • Gets the major incident box and delegates roles/gives out action cards | |
| • Assesses safety in the department and allocate a senior doctor to clear the department/contact bed manager to help with this | |
| Advises the following moves: | |
| • Informs the waiting room and asks people to go to minor injuries units (MIU) or go home and see GP/return tomorrow, etc. | |
| • Clears the remaining Minors patients to fracture clinic and explains there will be a long wait. Advises MIU or return tomorrow if able | |
| • Clears Majors patients to the wards | |
| • Clears Resus patients to ITU/theatre recovery/high dependency unit (HDU) | |
| • Locks down the department and sets up a triage area, usually by the paramedic entrance. All patients to enter by this triage area and be logged | |
| • Senior doctor to assess patients and categorise on arrival using a revised trauma score/triage sort tool | |
| P1: Immediate resuscitation/lifesaving treatment: will go to Resus beds/theatre/ITU | |
| P2: Urgent treatment, not immediately life-threatening: will go to Majors beds ± Minors | |
| P3: May have significant injuries: treatment can be delayed. Can go to fracture clinic/waiting room | |

| | |
|---|---|
| Sets up the department: Resus plus some of Majors will be additional Resus beds. Majors plus additional cubicles from Minors for the Majors patients. Minors and fracture clinic for the Minors patients | |
| Establishes where the control room is and senior management is on site, and establishes radio controls | |
| Considers a decontamination area: | |
| • Unknown chemical. Clarifies what the chemical is and what decontamination is occurring on scene | |
| • Sets up a decontamination area outside triage | |
| • Informs staff and use personal protective equipment (PPE) | |
| Informs and readies CT/theatres. Gets additional equipment ready | |
| Confirms understanding | |
| Asks if there are any further questions and closes the discussion | |

Total    /**33**

## Learning Points

If you have time, have a look at your own department's major incident plan. They are massive documents which you should not attempt to read the night before the exam or during an incident. Focus on summary documents, action cards, etc. Talk it through with your departmental major incident lead. The Hospital Major Incident Management and Medical Support (HMIMMS) is a useful course not only for the exam, but before your CCT.

The mark sheet above is a useful summary of the key elements of readying a department for a major incident—make sure you are aware of all these steps.

## 9.6 **Preparation for Inter-Hospital Transfer of Trauma Patient**

### Instructions for Candidate

You are the consultant in a trauma unit and wish to transfer a patient to your nearest major trauma centre (MTC), which is a 60-minute transfer by land. Please refer the patient (by phone) and make appropriate arrangements for the transfer. The case details are:

- A 24-year-old pedestrian hit by a car at 3 a.m. Arrived with GCS 12/15, with chest injury. He has had a trauma pan-CT and his injuries are:
  - ◆ Traumatic subarachnoid haemorrhage.
  - ◆ Right-sided flail chest: ribs 2 to 9 with a small pneumohaemothorax and pulmonary contusions.
  - ◆ Open fracture right wrist.
- Saturations are 94% on 15 litres/min $O_2$.
- HR 88, BP 123/78.
- Treatment: he has had 30 mg ketamine, 1 g tranexamic acid (TXA) IV, 1.2 g co-amoxiclav IV, and tetanus immunisation, and his wrist has been plastered.

You have an anaesthetic registrar available to transfer the patient.

### Mark Scheme Breakdown

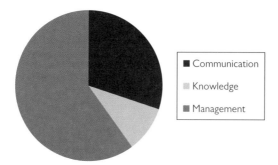

- Communication
- Knowledge
- Management

**Figure 9.6.1** Preparation for transfer mark scheme breakdown.

### Instructions for Actor

*Trauma Team Leader*

You are the receiving trauma team leader (TTL) at the MTC. Your ITU is currently full and will only accept the patient if it is clinically essential. You ask probing questions: does the patient really need to come here? If he is stable, can he be transferred in daylight hours? Accept the patient for transfer if given a good handover.

*Staff Nurse in Resus*

Ask the candidate what needs to happen now to get ready for the transfer.

# Instructions for Examiner

Observation only.

# Equipment Required

Patient details and a prompt card with the injuries listed.

# Mark Scheme

| | |
|---|---|
| Gathers information and checks the patient's details prior to making call | |
| Asks if any change to status of patient/suggests they would quickly review | |
| **Phone call:** | |
| Introduces self by name and grade, and states clearly where you are calling from | |
| States would like to transfer a trauma patient | |
| Gives a clear handover in a structured manner, e.g. ATMIST: | |
| • Age | |
| • Time of incident | |
| • Mechanism | |
| • Injuries/exam findings | |
| • Signs | |
| • Treatment given | |
| Gives a clear rationale for why the transfer is necessary. If probed: | |
| • Multiple body regions injured | |
| • Needs specialist input from cardiothoracics, neurosurgery, and orthopaedics/plastics | |
| • As per the trauma network guidance as multi-region injuries | |
| Decides about timing and mode of transfer (road vs air and explanation of choice), and escort | |
| Answers any questions from the receiving TTL and ends phone call | |
| Considers if further investigations or treatment is necessary prior to transfer | |
| Suggests using a transfer checklist | |
| Decision to transfer intubated with anaesthetic registrar | |
| Consideration of chest drain and nasogastric tube | |
| Ensures the case notes are copied and imaging is available | |

| | |
|---|---|
| Ensures the drugs required and fluids/blood products are available for transfer | |
| Considers neuroprotection | |
| Ensures the relatives are given details of the transfer and where to go | |
| Provides ETA for the receiving hospital on departure | |
| Books a blue light ambulance | |

Total    **/25**

# Learning Points

The main focus of this station is being able to give a succinct ATMIST for handover and readying the patient for transfer. Although many of you are unlikely to have to personally transfer a patient between hospitals, some of you who work in remote locations will do so. This scenario is also relevant to patients being transferred within the hospital, e.g. to CT or ITU, as similar thought processes and considerations are also required.

*Trauma Networks*

We recommend you familiarise yourself with your local trauma network policy.

## 9.7 **Colleague in Difficulty**

### Instructions for Candidate

One of the senior nurses has asked you to sort out a difficult situation. She has smelt alcohol on the breath of a doctor this morning and is concerned that she is dishevelled and has not been herself for a few weeks. Please investigate the matter and inform the doctor of how this will be managed.

### Mark Scheme Breakdown

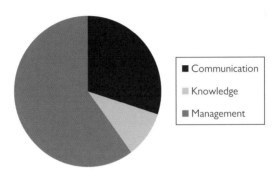

**Figure 9.7.1** Colleague in difficulty mark scheme breakdown.

### Instructions for Actor

You are Dr Harper. You have recently been going through a difficult time at home. Your husband left you a few months ago and you are now looking after your three children alone. The split is acrimonious, and you have been battling with your ex over financial support for the children. You have been drinking most nights as a result, and last night, after an argument, you had a bottle of wine and several glasses of gin and tonic. You drove to work this morning despite still feeling drunk. When confronted, you are tearful and scared of losing your job and your children.

### Instructions for Examiner

Observation only.

### Equipment Required

None.

# Mark Scheme

| | |
|---|---|
| Confirms with the nurse that patients are currently safe and no action is required | |
| Reassures the nurse you will deal with the situation and will review the SHO's work from today | |
| Agrees to feed back with the nurse after you have spoken with Dr Harper | |
| **Discussion with Dr Harper:** | |
| Introduces self and suggests talking to Dr Harper somewhere private | |
| Asks Dr Harper an open question, e.g. 'How are you?' | |
| Sensitively explains the concerns that have been raised | |
| If she does not volunteer information at this point, states concerned that she is not her usual self | |
| Explains that some errors have been made and you are worried something is wrong | |
| Allows her to talk and explain her concerns/what has been happening | |
| Responds sympathetically to Dr Harper's explanation | |
| Ask about specific difficulties that have led to this situation, e.g. family, home, health, money, stress, etc. | |
| Seeks information about the situation: frequency of drinking/ever driven or worked under the influence before | |
| Explains that patient safety is the priority and that she cannot work today | |
| Asks if she has any concerns about her patients or work today | |
| Ensures the patients are reviewed and handed over | |
| Checks when she is next due to work: suggests she takes some time off | |
| Asks if she recognises that this is a problem. Does she plan to engage to resolve the issue? | |
| Explains that you will need to inform her supervisor and the clinical lead | |
| Offers Dr Harper support. Suggests occupational health, her GP, or local alcohol services | |
| Asks about support from friends and family | |
| Considers the safety of her children: were they at home whilst she was drinking? Is there a safeguarding concern? | |
| Recognises that she will be unfit to drive home and suggests an alternative | |
| Explains that if she is dependent on alcohol, she should not be driving and should inform the DVLA and her insurance may be void | |

| | |
|---|---|
| Remains professional and non-confrontational throughout discussion | |
| Feeds back to the nurse that you have dealt with the situation and will ensure patient safety | |
| Summarises and closes discussion | |

Total    **/26**

## Learning Points

This case raises several issues regarding Dr Harper that need to be addressed: the safety of her patients, the safety of her children, and her own well-being. In addition, consider the impact this will have on the department, e.g. staffing and potentially impaired working relationships with colleagues. The gravity of the situation must be carefully balanced with providing support, with safety concerns as paramount. This is in line with the GMC's Good Medical Practice.

## Reference

https://www.gmc-uk.org/-/media/documents/good-medical-practice---english-20200128_pdf

## 9.8  **Complaint**

### Instructions for Candidate

You have received the following email from PALS and have agreed to phone the patient to discuss her concerns.

> 'I am writing to complain about the treatment I received in A&E when I attended with a deep cut to my thumb. I'd accidentally cut it with a knife 3 days earlier, but it was still really painful and I had some numbness and so wanted to get it checked out, as advised by 111. Your triage nurse was exceptionally rude and dismissive and said 'what do you want us to do with that? It is a healed cut? There is nothing to be done.' I was obviously very unhappy about this as I'd been directed there by 111, so I stayed to be seen. I was then assessed by a lovely nurse practitioner who was very kind and assessed me but said there was nothing wrong and just gave me some thumb exercises. The following week, I saw my GP as I still was in so much pain and they referred me to see plastic surgery, and I have since had to have emergency surgery to repair a nerve. They asked why I had waited so long to get it sorted and said I may have permanent damage.
>
> I am really angry about how I was spoken to by this nurse and I want her reprimanded, so no one else has to go through this.
>
> Yours sincerely,
>
> Anna Haworth'

### Mark Scheme Breakdown

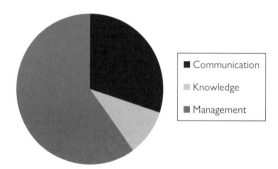

**Figure 9.8.1**  Complaint mark scheme breakdown.

### Instructions for Actor (via Telephone)

You remain really angry and your anger is directed at the triage nurse who you think was incompetent and rude and led the ENP to discount her symptoms. You still have some numbness after your digital nerve repair but do not want any further action taken against the ENP. You remain irate throughout the conversation and want the triage nurse to be fired. If this is not agreed, then you start shouting and threaten to submit a formal complaint to the Chief Executive.

## Equipment Required

None.

## Mark Scheme

| | |
|---|---|
| Introduces self to the patient | |
| Checks has the correct person on the phone | |
| Explains the call is in response to the PALS issue raised | |
| Clarifies concerns and the series of events | |
| Apologises for the perceived rudeness of triage nurse | |
| Apologises for the missed diagnosis | |
| Asks how the patient is doing now after her surgery | |
| States will ensure triage nurse is aware of complaint and inform her direct supervisor | |
| States will give feedback to the ENP in question | |
| Suggests will arrange teaching session for all the junior doctors and ENP in ED | |
| Stays calm and professional whilst the patient is verbally aggressive | |
| Does not make false promises or concede about reprimanding or sacking the nurse | |
| Attempts to diffuse the situation | |
| Advises her of formal complaint process | |
| Closes the conversation | |

Total    /**15**

## Learning Points

This station will test your skills in communication, de-escalation, and professionalism. This is a telephone conversation, so you cannot rely on the usual body language cues from the patient that would normally help you to respond and de-escalate any rising tensions. You must be sensitive to pauses in the conversation and to the volume and tone of voice. In turn, try to modulate your own voice and ensure that you speak clearly and calmly.

Become familiar with your hospital's complaints procedures and offer to signpost the patient, should they want to proceed with a complaint.

# Index

Tables and figures are indicated by *t* and *f* following the page number.

# X

X-rays
  acromioclavicular joint disruption  95*f*
  avulsion fracture of hip  98*f*
  cervical spine interpretation  169–71
  hand trauma  84*f*

mandibular fracture  126*f*
metaphyseal corner/bucket handle fracture  211*f*
Ottawa ankle and foot rules  72–3
paediatric elbow  140–4
Perthes' disease  230*f*
*see also* chest X-rays